BEING
SOBER

HARRY HAROUTUNIAN, MD

BEING
SOBER

A STEP-BY-STEP PLAN FOR GETTING TO,

GETTING THROUGH,

AND LIVING IN RECOVERY

REVISED AND EXPANDED EDITION

FOREWORD BY STEVEN TYLER

RODALE

NEW YORK

Copyright © 2021 by Harry L. Haroutunian, MD

Published in the United States by Rodale Books, an imprint of Random House, a division of Penguin Random House LLC, New York.

rodalebooks.com

RODALE and the Plant colophon are registered trademarks of Penguin Random House LLC.

Originally published in paperback in the United States by Rodale, an imprint of the Crown Publishing Group, a division of Penguin Random House LLC, New York, in 2013.

Library of Congress Cataloging-in-Publication Data is on file with the publisher.

ISBN 978-0-593-23623-9

Ebook ISBN 978-1-623-36006-1

Printed in the United States of America

Book design by Kara Plikaitis

Cover design by Kathleen Lynch/Black Kat Design

Cover photograph by Giuliano Del Muretto/Shutterstock

1 3 5 7 9 10 8 6 4 2

Second Paperback Edition

FOR MY WIFE, NICOLETTE, who is my foundation
and from whom I gain strength and conviction. She holds me to
a high standard, and I can only hope that all my efforts will never
disappoint her. And for my son, Aram. One of the greatest gifts
of this program is to see your own child embrace its principles, change
his life, and operate in the world as a principled participant.

Finish each day and be done with it.
You have done what you could. Some
blunders and absurdities have crept in;
forget them as soon as you can.
Tomorrow is a new day. You shall begin
it serenely and with too high a spirit to
be encumbered with your old nonsense.

—RALPH WALDO EMERSON

CONTENTS

ACKNOWLEDGMENTS

First and foremost, I would like to thank the people who were instrumental in getting this book to print—my brilliant agent, Linda Konner; Karen Chernyaev, who helped to piece the manuscript together; as well as Cheryl LaFlamme, for her untiring support and patience. Without them, this book might not have reached the electric and engaging folks at Rodale Inc., especially Ursula Cary.

In the addictions arena, it's important for me to acknowledge Terence Gorski; Rabbi Abraham Twerski, MD; Hazelden; and particularly the Betty Ford Center for their enormous contributions to the body of knowledge in the addiction field. To those beautiful people who supported me through those tough times: My gratitude can never be expressed to my nurse, Simone, who was with me for 25 years, or to the absolute saint Valery Yandow, MD, who was my mentor and guide during those early years of sobriety. Miki Boni, who, in a heartbeat, attended my Family Program at the Betty Ford Center when no one else could come, has always been my sister (even though we aren't truly related).

There are so many other people to thank—too numerous to list here—who are in my heart and my prayers on a daily basis. These are the ones who had the courage to say that something was wrong even when I could not listen and could not see. They all know who they are. They remain my closest and most trusted friends. I had some wonderful angels in my life to help me along the way, the heroes in my recovery. These are people to whom I owe my life.

And I can't leave out the men who began the program that saved my life. Because of Bill W. and Dr. Bob, founders of Alcoholics Anonymous, I learned that giving it up is the key, the missing part— the surrender that has brought me this windfall of grace. And, finally, to my beloved patients at the Betty Ford Center and the great patients of Vermont: We've shared our strengths and hopes together, getting through this thing one day at a time. I have so much gratitude toward all of you and for all that you've done for me.

FOREWORD

Dearest Harry,

It's with my deepest regret and heartfelt sorrow that, to the extent of the nature of the beast (addictions in general), I must tell you that I won't be getting high in the foreseeable future (except on my own bad ass) due to the Betty Ford Center and your one-of-a-kind experience, strength, and to-die-for hope, followed by an ancient teaching tool called Harry Har Har experiential hands-on psychological storytelling. My recovery is due exclusively to the Betty Ford Center, your friendship and words of wisdom, and, of course, my own trashed knees from repeatedly falling onto them.

Storytelling is an ongoing gift that helps me remember just how cunning the disease of addiction can be. One alcoholic or addict sharing his story with another is powerful medicine, and I've witnessed firsthand new alcoholic and drug-addicted people repeating phrases you spoke so eloquently at a lecture 24 hours prior. I believe that your storytelling alone, and the way you put your own passions into the storytelling, has helped thousands of Betty Ford Center alumni into quality years of sober life, and, oh yeah, I'm one of them.

Thanks, Harry.

Big love,
Steven Tyler

INTRODUCTION TO
THE SECOND EDITION

When *Being Sober* first came out in 2013, I was physician director of the professional and residential programs at the Betty Ford Center, where my work with the addicted was direct and hands on. I looked into their eyes, spoke with their families, and hugged them. We stayed in contact long after discharge. I've since retired from the Betty Ford Center, but I remain a part of many of my former patients' lives, and they remain a part of mine. The lives changed in treatment are not only the many celebrities we read about in the headlines but ordinary people from around the world. The recovery message is not exclusive but universal.

A lot has changed in my life since 2013. While I no longer work at the Betty Ford Center, I run my own addiction treatment practice with a focus on what I call "individualized treatment without walls." This model tends to each person's unique needs and delivers one-on-one attention for as long as necessary via today's technology and even good old-fashioned house calls. I'm still a firm believer in the Twelve Step Program and use it extensively in my practice. It is, after all, how I found and maintain recovery. But I'm now open to some less traditional approaches, including harm reduction and medications such as naltrexone to eliminate opioid and alcohol cravings. Addiction historian William White once said, "There are many pathways of long-term recovery, and all are cause for celebration." During this ongoing opioid epidemic, I couldn't agree more. People need help, and it's not for me to judge what form of help they will respond to best. In my current practice, the operative phrase is "meeting patients where they are at."

The purpose of this book is still threefold: to bring the heart of Twelve Step treatment to anyone struggling with addiction; to take you from despair to hope as you come to understand the healing phases of the disease; and to increase your loved ones' understanding of alcoholism and other drug addictions. Based on feedback from readers, I've added some content that expands the message concerning the ongoing opioid crisis, which had reached great heights during the first release of *Being Sober* but shows no sign of waning. I've also added a chapter on Emotional Sobriety and Advanced Recovery Topics. While you might not need to address these topics in early recovery, it's good to have a heads-up, as they will likely show up at some point down the road.

As in 2013, the disease of addiction affects about 1 out of 10 people in the United States, and in a culture that promotes alcohol and drug use, it is not going away anytime soon. Addiction is a chronic, organic, and fatal disease of the brain, responsible for untold damage to families, individual lives, and the economy. As baby boomers become the next crop of seniors with time on their hands, the disease will become even more prevalent.

Being Sober is written for those of you who need relief from an addiction lifestyle—whether for the first time or after umpteen stints in treatment. The book is also for you if you're in recovery but have either relapsed or feel a full-blown relapse coming on. If you are solid in your recovery, you will find in these pages a gentle reminder of why it is so important to stay on the recovery path. This book offers comfort and solutions—within these pages lies a $50,000 five-star treatment that has worked for thousands of people. My hope is that you will carry a dog-eared copy of this reference throughout your life as a source of serenity when times get hard and as a "how-to" book when recovery gets hard.

I can't think of a single person I've met who hasn't known someone close to them affected by the disease of addiction. We must break the cycle through education, which is why I wrote—and revised—this book. My hope is that even if you cannot or will not seek treatment, you can identify with the stories shared here and experience the promises and huge rewards of recovery.

In these pages, you will find the direction you need to get into and stay with a doable recovery plan. And you'll learn how to easily connect with others who are currently experiencing or have gone through the same things you are struggling with. It takes strength and courage to heal. I'll give you the tools you need to acquire that strength and courage, and then I'll take you further. I'll show you how to navigate meetings, tell you stories you'll be able to relate to, and share some important priorities. I will take you by the hand and get you started on a solid program of recovery. First, and perhaps most important, I will show you why addiction is not your fault.

CHAPTER 1

THE DISEASE OF ADDICTION

"Every day I thank God for inventing the blackout,
without which I would have drunk myself to death."

—ANONYMOUS

I DROVE HOME one cold November night through the mountains of Vermont. My moment of spiritual awakening came like Bill W.'s, the cofounder of Alcoholics Anonymous, who describes his moment of spiritual awakening in the form of a bright white light—only for me the light was blue and in my rearview mirror.

When the rookie cop got out of his patrol vehicle and walked up to my car, I thought I recognized him. He could have been a pediatric patient of mine, now grown up in jackboots and a Smokey hat. He told me that I had been wandering between the lines. I said, "Well, I thought that's where I was supposed to be—between the lines, that is."

I then did what any other red-blooded American alcoholic might do having the time, knowledge, and inclination: I blew out the side

1

of my mouth so his Breathalyzer test wouldn't work and so I could buy myself some time. On the way to the police station, I faked a hypoglycemic attack to bring out the entire rescue squad so they would become witnesses who could help explain my behavior. This would look good in court, I told myself.

Then I hired a detective. We went back to the scene of the crime and videotaped all the stripes on that highway and saw that some of those stripes wiggled and varied, a scenario that could give rise to the theory that it had only been an optical illusion that my car had been weaving. It also pointed to the possibility that the Vermont road crew who painted the lines was loaded at the time. As if that weren't enough, I hired a chemist to refute my blood alcohol level reading by explaining that at that temperature and at that time, in the middle of the night, and given the toothpaste I was using, all tests were, in all probability, invalid.

After examining the arrest record of this young cop, the detective and I determined he was probably a stalker who had followed many a bar employee home, stopping them and forcing them into DUI checks. I was just another victim. So we amassed a lot of evidence, and I spent a fortune because there was no way a guy like me was going to go down. I was a doctor with the gift of defiance and grandiosity, the perfect storm for an alcoholic.

We were preparing for trial when my lawyer said, "Hey, Doc, before we go to trial, would you like to see the videotape?"

"What videotape?"

"The videotape of your arrest that was made by the chief of police who was training the rookie cop. The chief, who's known you for 30 years and could have stopped the arrest, thought it was time you got a little help."

"Has anyone else seen this videotape?" I asked.

"Yes," he replied. "Just the state medical board and the district attorney."

A MATTER OF CHOICE?

We can define disease as a loss of function of an organ or organ system that produces a set of symptoms with a known or an unknown cause. For example, diabetes has a target organ, the pancreas. We know the cause, which is a dysfunction in insulin production or in insulin's action at the cellular level. And the effect is that the body becomes glucose intolerant, which results in high blood sugar levels that, over time, damage organs with small blood vessels, including the eyes, the kidneys, and the heart.

Type 1 diabetes is a chronic, lifelong, incurable disease that is absolutely treatable. A patient with diabetes follows dietary, exercise, and medication instructions to attempt to normalize blood sugar levels. But if left untreated, diabetes takes its toll on the body. Chronic elevated blood sugar levels cause the small blood vessels in the peripheral nerves, eyes, heart, and kidneys to thicken, eventually occluding proper bloodflow. This can result in pain, numbness, and tingling in the lower extremities; destruction in the retina; early susceptibility to heart attack; and, most especially, renal failure—the awesome consequences of a disease run rampant.

Are these consequences preventable? Often, the answer is yes. If the diabetic follows a daily treatment regimen, she can live to be 100. Left untreated, diabetes is a fatal disease. That is, it must be treated one day at a time. You don't get credit today for the insulin you took last week.

Multiple sclerosis (MS) is another example of a chronic, lifelong, fatal disease, treatable but not curable. The target organ system for MS is the brain and central nervous system. It is a chronic, organic disease of the brain with a relapsing and remitting pattern that may come and go with devastating symptoms.

For many years, alcoholism and drug addiction were considered a weak person's inability to control desire. Most people believed that drinking was simply a matter of choice and that anyone with a drinking or drug problem was reckless, self-absorbed, and irresponsible. Research dating back to the 1950s, however, has led most medical professionals, myself included, to understand that addiction is not a moral issue but a disease—a brain disease to be specific, and one that has genetic links. The National Institute on Alcohol Abuse and Alcoholism (NIAAA), the National Institute on Drug Abuse (NIDA), and the Substance Abuse and Mental Health Services Administration (SAMHSA) continue to do important research on the complex genetic disorder known as addiction.

We have proof. Addiction is a disease. So why do most people, including addicts and their family members, find this fact difficult to accept? Perhaps it's because addicts and alcoholics seeking their drug of choice have done some pretty bad things, transgressing the boundaries of society and the law. No doubt, an addict's behaviors can be intolerable. Living with an addict can bring family members to the brink of insanity.

But addiction is a brain disease with signs and symptoms manifested in part as behaviors. And like diabetes or MS, alcoholism and addiction have a target organ, a cause, and an effect, which we call symptoms.

THE TARGET ORGAN OF ADDICTION

The disease of alcoholism and drug addiction affects one of our more precious organs: the midbrain (more appropriately called the survival, or reptilian, brain), an area located just below the upper, or think-ing, brain. It is called the reptilian brain because it is the only brain that reptiles have and the only brain they have ever needed to survive for hundreds of millions of years. The midbrain dictates survival behaviors: to move away from danger and toward food; to breathe in and out; to eat and to rid the body of waste products; and, of course, to procreate. These survival behaviors require reinforcement so that they're repeated over and over again by generations to per-petuate the species. That reinforcement comes in the form of dopa-mine, a neurotransmitter that, when released by the brain, simply makes us feel great.

When we're parched, we seek water, knowing how good those first gulps of cool liquid will feel. When we experience orgasm through sexual intercourse, we're encouraged to procreate. These pleasurable feelings are directly related to the midbrain, which encourages us to repeat behaviors that feel good and to avoid those that don't.

Drugs of abuse affect the midbrain by causing it to release 2 to 10 times more dopamine than natural rewards do. If we're smoking or injecting our drug, the effects can be immediate and long lasting. At first, the "high" is bigger, better, and stronger than the natural high most of us get from pleasurable activities. Our brain rewards us for using drugs, and, drawn to the dopamine, we do it again and again.

Over time, our brain, overwhelmed by repeated surges in dopa-mine and other neurotransmitters, adapts. It either produces less dopamine or reduces the number of receptors that can receive dopamine signals. Our natural supply of dopamine plummets, and we have a hard time feeling pleasure from normal activities. At this point, we need to take drugs just to feel normal. If we want to feel the high we once felt, we need to take larger amounts of the drug than we first did—an effect known as tolerance.

The result is addiction, a condition that keeps us drinking and drugging even after our behavior has started to make us feel bad and negatively affect others.

THE CAUSE OF ADDICTION

Disease (excluding infectious disease) is often based on genetics, inherited traits passed down from generation to generation through DNA, and addiction is no exception. The disease of alcoholism and addiction is about 60 percent genetic; the other 40 percent is environmental. What do I mean by that? To experience addiction, we must first trigger the expression of our addiction genes. This is where environment enters the picture.

Even if we carry the addiction genes and drink or use drugs on occasion, we may never become addicted to drugs or alcohol. Someone who has inherited the genes and grows up in a healthy environment with little or no exposure to drugs and alcohol, and who doesn't experience any major traumatic life events, may never manifest the disease. Are they still genetically an addict or an alcoholic? Yes, they have those chromosomal traits. But the environment has not supported the disease's development. Conversely, someone with very little genetic contribution—three or four generations without a case of addiction or alcoholism in his family—who grows up living over a bar in an inner city, next to a crack house, and hanging out with a gang that's manufacturing methamphetamine and amphetamine has a pretty good chance of developing the disease of addiction primarily because of his environment.

One way to trigger addiction is to experience stress. Stress causes the adrenal glands to release the hormone cortisol. The stress could be good or bad—marriages or funerals, births or deaths, letters from the lottery commission or letters from the tax collector—it doesn't really matter. All events of significance will stimulate the release of cortisol, which has the effect of raising the dopamine requirements in the person who has the addiction genes—1 in 10 people in the United States.

Puberty, as luck would have it, is a stressor in and of itself. And we all go through it. Our bodies may differ from our peers in growth and maturity rates, causing us to feel awkward or like we don't belong. We may feel too young for this group and too old for that group. It's during this awkward, stressful stage that many of us are introduced to drugs or alcohol. When using for the first time, we may experience a warm glow or feel our inhibitions replaced by false courage. If we are among the 1 in 10 who are genetically predisposed to addiction, this can be a life-changing event—many alcoholics and addicts will tell you that the first time they had a sip of alcohol at age 12 or 14, they felt heavenly, normal, and comfortable in their own skin for the first time. We might not develop alcohol or drug addiction in these adolescent years or even in our twenties, but at some point in the future, under specific stressful circumstances, the relief of anxiety and discomfort through alcohol or drugs will be a remembered and welcome event.

The disease of addiction is very patient. Many who have had this type of euphoric experience with drugs or alcohol go through long periods of training, schooling, and employment where outside factors keep their disease at bay. The same people who say they will never drink before 5:00 p.m. or will never have a drink at lunchtime may find that when their life circumstances change due to financial difficulties, job loss, or the death of a spouse, the floodgates suddenly open. Even retirement can be a trigger: More and more people of retirement age find that their drinking or drugging patterns change dramatically when the structure and constraints of their work life are no longer present.

Once we establish high dopamine requirements, normal pleasures—a day with the kids, a beautiful sunrise, a painting, or good music—don't seem to satisfy the midbrain's requirements for reward. Something that has worked in the past, such as a surge of dopamine from alcohol, cocaine, methamphetamine, or an opioid, may serve the purpose.

I like to think of the carnival game where you hit a block with a big hammer, causing a weight to fly up a cable and ring a bell. Imagine that the bell being rung is a dopamine bell and ringing it on a regular basis is a requirement of survival. We have no choice. We must breathe. We must eat. And we must have reproductive activity to keep ringing the bell. Then a drug like cocaine comes along, causing a surge of dopamine that raises the bell 10 feet on the cable. Suddenly, the hammer, or those things that have caused pleasure in the past (good food, good sleep, sexual activity), isn't effective anymore. A bigger hammer is needed. Like heroin. Like opioids. Like cocaine. Like alcohol. The addictive substance trumps the normal behaviors that ring the bell and becomes a requirement for the bell ringing. In other words, our midbrain sends out cravings for the substance that it deems necessary for survival. The midbrain will require us to seek out the same substance, over and over and over again, until the cycle is broken.

THE SYMPTOMS OF ADDICTION

When we have a disease, we call certain traits symptoms, not behaviors. Addiction has its own list of physical symptoms, but it also claims a host of symptoms that affect behaviors. The symptoms of addiction are biological, emotional, social, and spiritual. In the field of addiction, we sometimes call them consequences.

Biological consequences (of alcohol). All drugs take a toll on the body, but alcohol affects you from head to toe.

- The brain may shrink or atrophy, like the brains of those with Alzheimer's disease. It's difficult to distinguish between the MRI of an Alzheimer's patient and the MRI of a chronic alcoholic. (Amazingly, brain damage caused by alcohol can often be reversed in recovery, and the brain regains its former size.)

- The digestive system becomes red or raw and may even bleed from the caustic effects of alcohol.

- Elevated liver enzymes give rise to fatty liver disease, which may progress to cirrhosis. The liver, shrunken and scarred from cirrhosis, causes a backup of bloodflow that results in varicose veins forming at the bottom of the esophagus, leaving the alcoholic more susceptible to internal bleeding. If internal bleeding does occur, the damaged liver is incapable of producing the blood-clotting factors it's responsible for, so there's nothing to stop the bloodflow. It's not uncommon for the terminal alcoholic to suffer a grotesque form of death—bleeding out through his mouth.

- The spleen becomes enlarged, which compromises the immune system by destroying valuable disease-fighting white blood cells. This increases the alcoholic's susceptibility to infection.

- The heart's muscular wall may thin and become flabby, causing the heart to overexpand and pump ineffectively, eventually leading to heart failure.

- High blood pressure, common in alcoholics, further damages the heart's effectiveness.

- The abdomen may swell with fluids that accumulate because of poor protein production by the liver.

- Heavy drinking may cause widespread joint pain. It's not uncommon for the hips to deteriorate, even in young adults, causing excruciating pain and requiring replacement.

- The alcoholic suffers from damage to the long nerves, causing skeletal muscle wasting in the extremities, severe neuropathic pain, and imbalance.

- Cognitive dysfunction, or an inability to think clearly, renders even brilliant men and women unable to figure out a grocery list or count their change when shopping. (Depression and anxiety also impair the alcoholic's ability to function.)

Biological consequences (of other drugs). Street drugs and prescription drugs used illegally come with their own set of issues.

- Overdose, whether from consuming too much of a drug, a lethal combination of drugs, or an impure drug, kills more than 70,000 people every year in the United States. (That's the same number of people who would die if two hundred 757s crashed this year and killed everyone on board.)

- Dirty needles used for injecting heroin, meth, and other drugs can carry deadly infections, especially HIV and hepatitis C, as well as cause skin infections and abscesses.

- Kidney disease, pulmonary complications, and liver disease are long-term consequences.

- All drugs have an effect on neurological connections and pathways in the brain, altering both structure and function, sometimes permanently.

- Stimulants such as amphetamines and cocaine increase heart rate, blood pressure, breathing rate, and core body temperature, sometimes to dangerous levels. Heart attacks are not uncommon among cocaine users.

- Snorting cocaine can produce a hole in the lining of the nose.

Social, emotional, and relationship consequences of alcohol and other drugs. Rifts begin to widen between parents and children, sisters and brothers, rendering the entire family dysfunctional in the presence of the active disease.

- Depression, anxiety, anger, isolation, and mood swings

- Poor performance at work or job loss

- Failing classes at school

- Loss of interest in hobbies or family events and activities

- Debt or financial ruin

- Family tension, arguments, and sometimes violence

- Divorce

- Legal consequences from DUIs or petty theft

- Enabling (loved ones providing money or support so the addict can continue to obtain his or her drug of choice)

- Loss of hope

- Loss of faith in the addict: "Maybe we would be better off without him."

Spiritual consequences. Using a chemical to deal with uncomfortable feelings, such as boredom or regret, separates us from having a relationship with ourselves and those we love. This is a seminal event that sets the disease in motion. When addiction is in full swing, we become obsessed with our drug of choice, the only thing in life that makes us feel anywhere near normal. The drug becomes more important than family and friends, and life becomes an endless cycle of using or drinking, or thinking about using or drinking. The emptiness creates a spiritual hole—a lack of hope and faith for any light at the end of the tunnel. "Why me, God?" we ask ourselves. "Maybe my family would be better off without me." But there is still a price of grave discomfort. We know we are detached from our soul, acting without integrity, and hurting those we love, but we cannot stop.

THE SHAME IN DISEASE

When I was about 6 years old, my father was diagnosed with tuberculosis. County administrators came, the nurses came, and soon my father was taken out of our house and transferred to a sanatorium, where the state required him to stay for 2 years. My mother said it was a place where his lungs would get healthy and he would be cured of his disease. I wondered why he couldn't get cured at home. When I asked, I heard: "Oh, we don't want anyone to catch it, so he has to go there."

Although we did not have the disease, once a month for about a year, my brothers and I had to stay home from Little League, football, playing army, or making a tree house with the neighbor kids. We had to get dressed up in that same shirt and tie that we wore to parochial school every day. But this was Saturday. And the wait was interminably long for that public health nurse to arrive at our house. I clearly remember it was like waiting for a monster to knock on our door—big nose, bad breath, scary, with a bag full of odd things. She wrapped something around my arm and pumped it up. Then she opened my shirt and listened to my chest. She examined me as if I weren't there. She would ask my mother, "Is he sweating at night?" "Does he have chills and fever?" "Have you seen any blood on his pillow?" "Does he have a cough?" "Is his weight stable?" Then she'd repeat the same invasive scenario with each of my brothers.

I know now what those visits were all about, but back then, one Saturday a month, I was treated as if I had tuberculosis. I didn't know what it was, but I knew it was the same thing that caused my dad to be ostracized and taken out of our home. I felt the shame.

The disease affected all of us.

JUST SAY NO?

I remember the day I heard First Lady Nancy Reagan suggest that everyone "just say no" to drugs. And I tried. I tried to say no and failed miserably. I felt different and apart from the norm. It made me think of myself as a broken person who had not learned to live in a society ruled by dignity and courage. No matter how hard I tried, I could never just say no; I felt shame.

When I learned that the area of the brain affected by this fatal disease is the same area from which emanates my heartbeat, my next breath, and all my vital functions, I finally understood that I could no more say no to that next drink than I could say no to that next breath.

THE DIFFERENCE BETWEEN CHOICE AND DISEASE

Am I responsible for my inheritance? My height, eye color, or gender? My propensity to develop MS or diabetes? If someone has diabetes, do we put that person in prison?

Alcoholics and drug addicts are often accused of choosing their fate, but there is little free will involved in addiction, just as there is no free will involved when someone is diagnosed with type 1 diabetes. Addicts simply cannot turn off the brain's natural desire for dopamine.

I have never heard an alcoholic say to his family, "Good night. I'm going out. Save a little cash for my bail money. I plan to have my fifth DUI tonight." No, that's never the plan. The plan is to be able to control alcohol or drugs and to avoid legal consequences, but it just doesn't work that way. For the person with the genetic propensity to develop addiction, the first drink is a choice. The first shot of heroin is a choice. But addiction is not a choice. Addiction is *not* a choice—it's a disease with a target organ, a cause, and a set of symptoms. It is chronic and organic. It relapses. It remits. It is cunning, baffling, and powerful, but, if addiction is treated one day at a time, lasting recovery is the promise for each and every alcoholic or addict. All that is required is the willingness to take the first steps. One of the very first steps is abstinence.

Your brain is no dummy. It quickly learns that the drug will ring the bell. It sets up cravings in the form of chemicals in the brain that will perpetuate this survival response. The drug then becomes the new coping mechanism for stress. After a period of abstinence, however, the ball falls down to its original position and our dopamine requirements are reset. We no longer require the surge of dopamine that was produced by our drug of choice, and in early recovery we see the return of pleasure and reward from the normal things—good food, a day in the park, soothing music, a first communion, or a bar mitzvah.

A CLOSER LOOK AT CHOICE

If addiction is not a choice, then what is? When I make a choice, I use my upper brain—the part of the brain responsible for making decisions. Let's say I see someone with a really nice watch. In the past, I used to have a watch like that, and boy, I'd like to have one now. I see an opportunity to snag it from a jewelry store when no one is looking. I'm also feeling deprived, so I'm justifying my projected infraction. If I get away with it, at least I'll have the watch; if I don't, well, I won't be put in jail for life for a stolen watch. So I make the decision. *Pow!* I grab the watch, slide it into my pocket, and walk quickly out of the store.

What made me do it? I've never stolen anything before. I'm not overly materialistic and wouldn't call myself compulsive. Perhaps I have some health or behavioral issues—I'm antisocial or have poor impulse control. Or perhaps I felt deprived and had bad parental examples who never taught me to control my greed. But in the end, it was a bad choice, and I am at fault. I am responsible for those actions.

I am not addicted to watches. It was free will. I can stop this behavior. It was a conscious choice. This type of decision making takes place in a different section of the brain than addiction does. Location. Location. Location.

A DISEASE BY ANY OTHER NAME

I have the disease of arthritis. Some days it is very symptomatic. I wake up to pain in my knees and back, and I know a hot shower will help. Or a light workout in the gym. Maybe even a hot tub. And certain medication—an aspirin or ibuprofen—will go a long way toward keeping the symptoms that I inherited from my family at bay.

I also have the disease of alcoholism. Some days it is symptomatic. It reminds me that it is still in my life despite the fact that it's been a long time since I've had a drink. It expresses itself first by unawareness and by denying that it exists. Then I go on and misbehave. I can become willful and filled with self-pity, arrogance, or grandiosity. I can be fearful and doubtful. I can lack courage and want to give up my will to persevere or pursue certain goals. I can sink into shame and avoid accountability. I can harbor resentment and anger and plot and defy. Or, I can reach for medication. I pick up the phone and call another person with the disease who understands how I feel. I say a prayer and ask for help. I go to a meeting with a bunch of other people who have this disease and listen to their stories, and I don't feel so different, so victimized. This is the aspirin, or the ibuprofen, for the disease of addiction. I reach out to another and ask for help.

I'm happy to become accountable and await the gifts that appear as my symptoms subside. I become more agreeable. I laugh like hell. I get a smattering of dignity. I call my son. I look into my wife's eyes, smell the roses, and look to the sky in gratitude.

———

MY LAWYER PLAYED the videotape of my arrest. I saw what I did and didn't like it. I wasn't a sloppy drunk; I was arrogant. It wasn't me.

But what scared me the most was that on the ride to the police station, I had no idea that the chief of police was in the car with the rookie. The whole time I was blacked out.

My attorney then produced a pamphlet for the Vermont Practitioner Health Program, which had been given to him by an investigator in the state attorney general's office. Apparently, health professionals who get charged with DUIs are reported to the attorney general's office, and the state medical board gets involved. I had seen this pamphlet before. Countless copies of it had arrived at my office in mailings from the Vermont Medical Society offering help to any physician in trouble with drugs or alcohol, but I had just discarded them.

I felt as if I had tumbled to the bottom of a rock pile. I contacted the people at the health program, found an addiction treatment specialist, dismissed the lawyer who would no longer be needed to fight the charges, and made arrangements to finally get some help for a disease that had been manifesting itself at various times since I was a teenager. I made arrangements to have my practice covered and pleaded guilty in court to charges that had been reduced to reckless endangerment. I lost my driver's license for 30 days, paid my fine, went to classes, and learned about driving while under the influence and the body's metabolism of alcohol—information I had forgotten since medical school or simply was never taught.

Then, in my inimitable alcoholic fashion, I went out and got drunk. I drank for about another year just to solidify the diagnosis so there would be no doubt that, despite adverse consequences, I would persist in doing what I always did and get the same result.

That videotape is in my safe now, and I watch it every year on the anniversary of my sobriety.

— TAKEAWAYS —

» Science has proven that addiction is a brain disease.

» Addiction is triggered by genetics and/or environment.

» Like other diseases, addiction has a target organ, a cause, and a set of signs and symptoms.

» Addiction has biological, emotional, social, and spiritual consequences.

» Although using drugs or alcohol for the first time is almost always a choice, addiction is not a choice but a disease.

CHAPTER 2

BUT I'M NOT A FALLING-DOWN DRUNK!

"A boo is a lot louder than a cheer."

—LANCE ARMSTRONG

WHEN I WAS still a medical student, most of my friends already called me Doc, and I was the go-to person, or "anchor man," during times of sickness or trouble. One particular day, I got a frantic phone call from a couple of friends who said, "Harry, you gotta get over to Jake's house. He just got back from Mexico, and something's very wrong."

Jake had walked into his empty house and found that his wife had left him with nothing. He was shocked, literally, when he tried to switch on the lights and found that the switch plates were missing. The showerhead and the faucets were gone too, along with the shower curtain, rod, and rings. Even the little cap that covers the garbage disposal was missing. Everything. Mercifully, she did leave the toilet handle; otherwise, the apartment was stripped bare.

Jake was bright yellow, jaundiced from some sort of hepatic or liver failure. He was as sick as a dog. His friends recognized it immediately and called me. I found him lying on a makeshift cot brought in with some blankets and a pillow. "Good God, Jake," I said. "What have you done to yourself?"

Jake's drawn-out reply was "Quaa-a-a-a-ludes."

"And how many Quaaludes did you take?" I asked.

"F-f-f-f-forty," he managed to reply.

I knew that Quaaludes were easy to obtain in Mexico.

"Forty Quaaludes?" I asked. "Why?"

His response: "Gee, I don't know, they were only a buck apiece."

Now that's alcoholic and addictive thinking. Take as much as we can or more. More. We have the disease of more. (Jake's yellow and red lights were broken; he only saw green lights.)

There, but for the grace of God, go I.

ABUSE OR ADDICTION?

Jake's addiction was easy to spot. Jake couldn't stop with just one Quaalude—he had to take a life-threatening dose. Jake's wife left him because of his using, communicating her anger by taking everything possible from his physical world. Jake suffered physical consequences because of his using—he had liver disease and almost died of an overdose. It doesn't take a professional addiction counselor to understand that Jake was an addict. But for Jake, the realization didn't come so easily. He only saw the green light when it came to consuming drugs. For the alcoholic or addict whose life circumstances are not as extreme as Jake's, the realization comes even harder.

At the Betty Ford Center, we only made the diagnosis of alcoholism or drug dependence. We never called anyone an alcoholic or an addict until he or she first had that self-revelation. Once a person identified as an alcoholic or addict, then that permission was granted to us. So, before we go any further, let's take a look at the various levels of use and decide where you or your loved one falls on the spectrum.

Not everyone who drinks is an alcoholic. Not everyone who uses illicit drugs is an addict. By the same token, not every alcoholic is a falling-down drunk and not every drug addict is wandering the streets. So how do we tell if we've crossed the line into addiction?

Social or Occasional Drinker

Some people can "take it or leave it." They might have a drink or two at a wedding or a nice dinner, but they don't get intoxicated and don't think about alcohol again for months or until the next big social event. This person is usually not at risk for becoming an addict.

Problem Drinker/User

The problem drinker/user is at risk. They consume alcohol or drugs regularly with occasional periods of intoxication. Although problem drinkers/users may "grow out of it," such as the college student who parties a lot in school but becomes more of an occasional drinker when the responsibilities of a job and family enter the picture, chances are good that there's trouble afoot.

Abuser

The abuser's regular consumption of alcohol or drugs is now identified by friends, family, and coworkers as a problem that also affects them.

Alcoholic/Addict

The relationship with alcohol or drugs has progressed fully. This person is experiencing biological, psychological, social, and spiritual consequences. He or she cannot stop. The pattern may be episodic bingeing or regular consumption, but the result is always unpredictable.

THE QUESTIONNAIRE

Online, you can probably find a hundred different questionnaires that can help you determine whether you might have a problem with drugs or alcohol. Although not conclusive, a self-assessment is a good place to start. More thorough evaluations are available, everything from a brief phone conversation with a counselor to a 7-day clinical diagnostic evaluation. But for now, answer this questionnaire, which is found on the Betty Ford Center website and has been reprinted here with permission.

YOUR "YES" ANSWER TOTAL:

One "YES" answer:

> Be aware. You may have or you may develop a problem with alcohol or other drugs.

Two or more "YES" answers:

> Indicates you have problems with alcohol and/or drugs and should seek help immediately.

Do you have a problem with alcohol or other drugs?

Questions		YES	NO
1.	Do you drink or use to overcome shyness or to feel more confident?		
2.	Are you having money troubles because of drinking or using?		
3.	Do you ever stay home from work because of drinking or using?		
4.	Is drinking or using causing trouble in your family?		
5.	Is drinking or using giving you a bad reputation?		
6.	Have you lost a job or a business because of drinking or using?		
7.	Do you drink or use to escape your problems?		
8.	Do you drink or use when you are alone?		
9.	Do you have blackouts? (Loss of memory for events that happened or of actions you performed while drinking or using?)		
10.	Do you feel remorse after drinking or using?		
11.	Do you need a drink at a definite time every day?		
12.	Do you drink in the morning?		
13.	Have you ever been in a hospital because of drinking or using?		
14.	Has a doctor ever treated you for your drinking or using?		
15.	Do you drink or use too much at the wrong time?		
16.	Do you make promises to yourself or others about your drinking or using?		
17.	Do you have to keep on drinking or using once you have started?		
18.	Is drinking or using making it hard for you to sleep?		
19.	Have you had an accident because of drinking or using?		
20.	Do you drink or use to relieve the painfulness of living?		
21.	Do you have trouble disposing of cans or bottles?		
22.	Are you less particular about people you are with and the places you go when you are drinking or using?		
23.	Have you been arrested more than once for drunk driving or driving under the influence of drugs?		
24.	Has drinking or using affected your health?		

Reprinted with permission from www.bettyfordcenter.org.

If, based on your answers to the questionnaire, you believe you're not addicted, feel free to carry on as usual. You might, though, want to continue reading to the end. (There was a reason you picked up this book in the first place, right?) You may learn something new about yourself and about addiction. If you answered yes to two or more questions, you're "borderline" addicted, or you can't be sure you answered the questions honestly, please read on. What follows may surprise you.

THE FIVE STAGES OF CHANGE

Most things have a tipping point—the point at which the buildup of small changes causes enough momentum to create a big change. In coming to terms with the idea that we might be alcoholics or addicts, many of us go through a similar process. We make small changes in how we think and act, and once we've gone through our process, the momentum carries us the rest of the way.

About 25 years ago, James Prochaska, PhD, and Carlo DiClemente, PhD, two researchers at the University of Rhode Island, were trying to figure out the process smokers went through to quit nicotine. They came up with the now famous Stages of Change Model. Dr. Prochaska and Dr. DiClemente determined that addicts go through five stages of change before quitting their drug of choice.

Telling a person they need to change falls on deaf ears unless that person is ready to hear it. The five stages addicts and alcoholics go through when they're ready to make a change are (1) precontemplation, (2) contemplation, (3) preparation/determination, (4) action/willpower, and (5) maintenance. How long we stay in each stage is up to us. It's possible to go through all five stages in the course of a day. It's also possible to take two steps forward and one step back. As you read through the five stages, consider which stage you might be in right now.

STAGE ONE: Precontemplation

In the precontemplation stage, we are in denial. We aren't thinking seriously about changing. We don't want to listen to others tell us we need to change. We're typically defensive and don't view our drinking or using as a problem.

STAGE TWO: Contemplation

The contemplation stage involves awareness. We are aware that our drinking or using is causing some consequences. In this stage, we're doing our own risk/benefit analysis. We're not completely convinced that giving up our drug of choice is worth it, although we can imagine that there are some benefits. Many addicts and alcoholics never get beyond this stage. We continue to look for excuses or others to blame for the consequences of our actions while under the influence.

STAGE THREE: Preparation/Determination

In Stage Three, we're committed to the idea of making a change. We know we have to do something, and we are determined to figure out what it is we need to do. We call clinics, read books (such as this one), or talk to people in recovery. We need solutions. We've accepted that we need to change.

STAGE FOUR: Action/Willpower

If we've done our research in Stage Three, we're usually more successful in Stage Four, when we go beyond commitment. Now we believe we can change, and we take an active role in making a change. For most people, Stage Four is fairly brief (it can last anywhere from 1 hour to 6 months). We review our commitment and take steps to implement our plan. At this stage, we are open to receiving help.

STAGE FIVE: Maintenance

In Stage Five, our goal is to maintain abstinence. We are patient with ourselves and remind ourselves that our goal is worthwhile. We can anticipate situations that could trigger relapse, and we have a prevention plan in place.

LOSING A BEST FRIEND

Even though the writing may be on the wall and everyone around us can see we have an issue, many of us hold on to the notion that we can continue to drink or use without consequences. We do this because our whiskey, Valium, or heroin has become a good and reliable friend, always able to make us feel better, at least at first. Saying we're an addict or alcoholic means giving up that friend, and where does that leave us? Alone, afraid, and miserable.

Yet deep down we know that our good friend has also done us wrong. It has betrayed us and tricked us into believing that if we chased it long enough, it would continue to bring us relief. But we come to realize that we won't ever experience the euphoria we felt when we first

THE CONTINENTAL ALCOHOLIC

One of my favorite parts of *Alcoholics Anonymous* (aka the Big Book) is "More About Alcoholics," which lists all of the tricks of the trade that alcoholics have used to adjust their drinking habits: switching from wine to beer, or from beer to wine, or from light beer to mixed drinks after 5:00 p.m. and only on weekends; abstaining for Lent, when going on vacation, or when not on vacation.

I had the idea that I only had continental alcoholism. Continental alcoholism, of course, is only active in the continental United States. That meant that if I were lucky enough to befriend an Inuit or other Alaskan, or to visit Hawaii, I might have been granted a reprieve. And while on the European continent or anyplace else in the world? I was absolutely a new man.

I had many opportunities to disprove my theory. I disproved it in France. I disproved it in Italy. I disproved it in Nepal. I disproved it in Hawaii. I never really got to disprove it in Alaska, but I certainly got to disprove it in the Caribbean Islands, in Mexico, and, of course, in the airplanes that took me to all those different places. I guess my theory of continental alcoholism didn't really hold much water, or any liquid capable of intoxicating a brain such as mine.

used our drug of choice. Because of how the pleasure pathways in the brain work, that euphoria is long gone—the dopamine bell was raised long ago. In desperation, and because we don't know what else to do, we return to our drug of choice in hopes of finding relief.

Interrupting the pattern and making real change takes honesty, courage, and surrender. It also means grieving the loss of our best friend.

YOU ARE NOT ALONE

According to SAMHSA's National Survey on Drug Use and Health, 21.2 million people age 12 or older—7.8 percent of that population—needed treatment for an illicit drug or alcohol abuse problem in 2018, but only 2.4 million of those who needed treatment received it at a specialty facility. That tells us that, in all likelihood, about 19 million people in the United States are walking around with addiction and not getting help for it.

Addiction spans all walks of life—the young, old, professional, jobless. Your neighbor, your boss, your doctor, your favorite actor—any one of them could have a problem with alcohol or drugs. (We like to say that addiction is an equal opportunity destroyer.) Most people do a pretty darn good job of hiding it, at least for a while.

The bottom line is this: You are not alone. In addition to the 21 million people you could be sharing a room with at a treatment center, there are millions of people in the world who are in recovery or living a life of sobriety, free of alcohol and drugs.

SHAME, SHAME, SHAME

In Chapter 1 we discussed the fact that addiction is a disease. For some people, this knowledge alone is enough to strip away any feelings of shame about addiction. We are not bad people; we just have some bad genes. Still, the old stereotype of addiction as a moral failure has not disappeared. We may even harbor some of our own harsh opinions about addicts and alcoholics, becoming our own worst enemy. More troublesome to us may be knowing that we've done some things while drunk or high that we now regret, things that go against our personal moral code.

Shame is the feeling that *I am something bad (and others know it)*. Shame is different from guilt, which is the feeling that comes from thinking *I did something bad, and I know it*. Shame has the power to make us feel worthless and inadequate; it's the opposite of self-worth. Shame is an overwhelming negative emotion, and it prevents us from being able to fully love and appreciate ourselves. Shame is powerful *and* smart. It is capable of disguising itself as isolation, arrogance, anger, and aggressiveness. And deep, buried shame causes us to act out at the most inappropriate of times and then to blame others for our behavior. This is shame at its best.

Even though addiction is a disease, most of us feel shame in being an addict or alcoholic. Either we don't realize it's a disease, others imply or tell us outright that we're worthless because of our drinking or using, or we do some shameful things (such as stealing money or pills from our grandmother) that make us feel bad about ourselves. Some of us carry shameful feelings from childhood and use drugs or alcohol to bury those feelings.

Feeling guilty can sometimes be good only because it gets us to feel remorse and behave better the next time or to correct whatever we did that was wrong. Shame, on the other hand, serves no purpose. It makes us feel "less than" others, less than who we are. Nobody wins when we feel shame. To come to terms with addiction, we need to be able to recognize and eliminate feelings of shame.

THE MANY FACES OF SHAME

Answer the following questions honestly, using a scale of 1–5
(1 = strongly disagree; 5 = strongly agree):

A. ___I take care of myself.

B. ___People who get their hair and nails done and who go to
the doctor and dentist are selfish.

A. ___I make sure to exercise and eat healthy meals.

B. ___People who belong to health clubs and are always
talking about weight are self-absorbed.

A. ___I deserve to be treated well by others.

B. ___Most people are mean, evil, or untrustworthy.

A. ___I deserve the nice things in life.

B. ___The world is full of greedy and selfish people.

A. ___I accept compliments easily.

B. ___I should be punished for my behavior.

Add up the A points and add up the B points. If the A score is
higher than the B score, you are probably feeling pretty good about
yourself. If the B score is higher than the A score, you may be feeling a
lot of shame, and you may be projecting, or transferring feelings about
yourself that you can't accept onto others.

Try This: Listen closely to your thoughts and to how you talk
to others. Whenever you find yourself tempted to think or say
something negative about someone such as "He's selfish," ask yourself whether the same could be true of you. Be rigorously honest. If
the answer is "yes," make a point to accept that you might sometimes behave selfishly—then forgive yourself.

ADMIT VERSUS ACCEPT

Picture this: You are in a deep well, and you have a ladder and a shovel. Do you want to climb out, or must you dig deeper? Knowing what we know now about addiction, if we're addicted, we can safely admit it. We can say to ourselves, "My name is _____, and I am an alcoholic/addict." Once we identify as an addict and fully accept our disease, we can change. Admitting it is one thing. Accepting it takes us to another level—it moves us from Stage Two to Stage Four or Five in a heartbeat.

Great people have turned their lives around by accepting with humility the presence of the disease in their lives. If they can do it, you can, too. We must believe that we are worth the treatment needed to get well. Punishment does not work. Stop beating yourself up.

We know from the statistics that addiction isn't going away. Millions of people are in recovery and that number continues to grow, but every generation brings with it another 10 percent of the population that will most likely become addicted at some point in their lives because of their genetics and/or the environment in which they live.

This tells us three things: (1) You are not alone; (2) There's no shame in being an alcoholic/addict; and (3) There's no reason not to get help. You've taken an important step by picking up this book and opening it to the first page. All you have to do is keep reading, and you will be on your way to a rewarding life of recovery.

— TAKEAWAYS —

» Not everyone who drinks is an alcoholic; and not every alcoholic is a falling-down drunk.

» We can cross the line from problem drinking/using into addiction.

» Questionnaires or clinical evaluations can help us determine whether we have an addiction.

» To change addictive behavior, we typically go through five stages.

» Most addicts and alcoholics carry around a lot of shame, a negative emotion we can do without.

» Acceptance leads to change.

CHAPTER 3

THE HIGH-
FUNCTIONING
ADDICT

*"As a surgeon you have to have a controlled arrogance.
If it's uncontrolled, you kill people, but you have to be
pretty arrogant to saw through a person's chest, take out
their heart, and believe you can fix it. Then, when you
succeed and the patient survives, you pray, because it's
only by the grace of God that you get there."*

—MEHMET OZ, MD

DAVE WAS AN accomplished surgeon. Like many successful professionals, he was proud of his work and spent way too many hours at the
hospital. And why not? This was where he received positive feedback
and his sense of self-worth. Although a good husband and father to a
newborn, Dave really only identified as a doctor. He celebrated his time
off with great abandon and a great deal of alcohol. One day Dave was

feeling some pain and decided to try an opioid. For him it was alcohol in pill form. His pain disappeared and so did his anxiety. He felt calm and relaxed, and he was sleeping better at night. Soon the pills led to patches, which led to injections. Before long, Dave found himself addicted to a powerful narcotic called fentanyl. Only now, instead of taking it to calm his nerves, he used it to avoid feeling withdrawal symptoms. Dave was using fentanyl daily just to feel normal.

At the height of his disease, Dave unwittingly picked up the wrong syringe, took it into the hospital bathroom, and injected himself. He fell to the floor. His face pressed against the cold terrazzo tile, he looked out from under the stall doors, across the empty room, and knew intuitively what had happened. His eyes, the only part of him that could move, managed to see that he had injected himself with a paralytic agent. In a matter of seconds, his respiratory muscles would be paralyzed and, unless he got help, he'd be dead. In that brief second, Dave's life passed before his eyes. He heard himself gasping for air and then in one dramatic moment, air rushed into his lungs. The very quick-acting drug had worn off, and he began to breathe again. He stood up, washed himself at the sink, straightened out his scrub suit, went into the OR, and meticulously did the next procedure.

That night, scared to death, Dave told his wife what happened and described the fear that gripped him as he lay paralyzed on the floor. He resolved to get rid of every pill in the house and to never do drugs again. He ran through the house gathering up all the pain prescriptions and any other medications he could find. He proceeded to dump all of the pills into the baby's diaper pail and was overcome with relief knowing that it was all over.

At 4:00 a.m. his wife awoke, somewhat startled. She realized that Dave was not in the bed, so she went downstairs. She gasped in horror at what she saw. There, kneeling on the floor, over the open diaper bucket, was the esteemed surgeon reaching into the soiled water, desperately searching to retrieve any pill that was not yet dissolved.

I often refer to addiction as an equal opportunity destroyer. Addiction knows no boundaries. Who you are, what you know, how much you own—it all carries little weight with this cunning and baffling disease. Indeed, some people get into recovery at the point when they are homeless, living off the streets, searching Dumpsters, and at the brink of absolute, incomprehensible demoralization. But there are also addicts and alcoholics who arrive at a crossroads because of their success—and the feelings of entitlement that accompany their accomplishments.

I'm talking about the high-functioning, high-achieving alcoholic or addict, a special case worthy of an intense and very specific approach to recovery. Whole programs are devoted to this group. The high-achieving group includes physicians, attorneys, pilots, executives, professional athletes, and entertainers—people who, because of their legacy, accomplishments, and success, tend to find it much more difficult to embrace the qualities of surrender and connected spirituality that will get them into a safe recovery.

Those who fall into this category face a particularly tough road, and getting them to accept help can seem next to impossible. If they are not forced into treatment by a court, a professional board, or their employer, they are best helped by a professional intervention. Afterward, they typically enter lengthy inpatient treatment. But there are many paths to recovery, including long-term outpatient treatment tailored to the high achiever's specific needs. The good news is that, once they've accepted recovery, high achievers have the greatest chance of staying in it.

NOT AT FAULT

The phrase "They are not at fault" comes from the beginning of Chapter 5 in *Alcoholics Anonymous* (aka the Big Book), which was first published in 1939 to help spread the word about Twelve Step recovery. It states, "Rarely have we seen a person fail who has thoroughly followed our path. Those who do not recover are people who cannot or will not completely give themselves to this simple program, usually men and women who are constitutionally incapable of being honest with themselves. There are such unfortunates. They are not at fault; they seem to have been born that way. They are naturally incapable of grasping and developing a manner of living which demands rigorous honesty. Their chances are less than average."

High achievers are often part of this group, if only because they have been so highly successful in creating a system they can use and abuse to keep themselves in their addiction. A system might look something like working 15-hour shifts to ensure they've earned the "reward" that comes at the end of that shift. Recognizing that this system exists is the rigorous honesty that's required of the high achiever.

High-achieving addicts and alcoholics are masters at using their talents, in their specific and chosen professions, to attempt to control the substances they use. Pilots, so adept at controlling their craft and managing dozens of instruments, flight plans, control towers, and passenger safety, are confused when they find out they can't control alcohol or drugs in the same way. Physicians, with all of their academic and physiologic knowledge, try to know their way around the disease of addiction by explaining the brain's intricate neuropathways and by tweaking doses of self-prescribed medications in a dance of manipulation that eventually ends in some catastrophe. Lawyers use their well-practiced talent of argument to argue their way around the diagnosis.

It's no wonder that these professionals have their own Twelve Step recovery groups: the Caduceus meeting for physicians, the Other Bar group for attorneys, and Birds of a Feather for pilots. In these specialized meetings, high achievers can see and present themselves as alcoholics and addicts first and as doctors, lawyers, and pilots second. Here men and women safely share the unique circumstances surrounding their addiction and the powerful atmosphere of their careers.

THE COVER-UP

High-achieving professionals who have the disease of addiction usually have systems firmly in place to keep the diagnosis and detection of their disease at bay.

In the Workplace

Busy professionals often entrust their calendar, finances, and work and leisure schedules to a trusted office manager. This support is invaluable, helping to jockey office hours, hospital meetings, surgical schedules, conferences, court dates, deadlines, or travel arrangements. In turn, support people also depend upon the professional for their own livelihood and have a great vested interest in establishing a rigid and high pedestal upon which they place their employer. Any attempt to assail that pedestal is seen, by the high achiever, as a hostile attempt. So support staff members—those who are most privy to their boss's comings and goings—easily get wrapped up in the defensiveness and denial that is the hallmark of the disease of addiction. These folks are often the deflectors of inquiry, the explainers of abnormal behavior, and the excuse makers:

"The doctor was on call very late last night."

"Sorry he showed up late; his beeper failed."

"His speech was slurred? You just woke him out of a sound sleep."

"I'm sorry. The counselor has been studying all night preparing a large brief. Missing that appointment was quite understandable given his busy schedule."

In the Home

For the addicted professional, home life often falls apart before career, but usually this disruption is kept quiet, hidden from the public. Spouses, accustomed to a high standard of living, fear financial and social repercussions. The thought pattern is usually the same: *If I expose my spouse's addiction, he or she will lose a highly coveted position, economic security, respect, reputation, social status, and friends.* In other words, the family's entire world would change and the spouse would go down with the addict or alcoholic. The thought of airing such dirty laundry to a wide audience—patients, fans, or clients, whose respect the professional has earned—is unimaginable.

Children sense that Mom or Dad is beyond reproach. They sense the shame in a household and feel burdened by the presence of addiction, thinking that somehow they are to blame. They certainly feel the effects of parental isolation and anger and are no strangers to resentment of their own. Their sense of abandonment may translate to poor performance in school or acting-out behaviors in general.

By the time the high-functioning patient seeks help, usually major disruption has taken place in the home. The kids may have grown up surrounded by lies and dysfunction. They may be dealing with the emotional consequences of having an absentee dad or mom. Wealthy, high-achieving families are not immune to anger, violence, abuse, or abandonment, but they do have strong incentives to cover it up. Eventually, family relationships deteriorate, which can lead to separation and divorce proceedings.

EXPOSURE

As the disease of addiction progresses, the high-functioning addict starts to misbehave in public. Bills are left unpaid. Coworkers and neighbors start to whisper and circulate innuendos. Public intoxication and driving violations follow, and the next tree to fall after family is professional status in the community. The last bastion is typically the all-protected workplace.

I've seen far too many physicians divorced and living alone in despair and economic ruin suit up and show up each day for work, protected by loyal staff members who have worked with them for years. The system works until finally a patient complaint, a behavioral issue, or a mistake in the operating room brings the physician's addiction to the attention of hospital administrators.

"Support" systems at home and work are often responsible for delaying the diagnosis of addiction in the professional for many years. The disease goes underground, and only after smoldering and festering below the radar does it begin to appear and get noticed at a very advanced stage, with pronounced physical, psychological, and social consequences. Convincing the reluctant professional that there's a problem usually requires some effort, even physical proof—a diagnostic evaluation, forensic data (such as hair analysis), and prescription records. Even then, sometimes only the threat of losing licensure, social status, or employment can convince the professional to enter treatment—a treatment that is usually long and intense.

TOO SMART TO SEEK HELP

I've never met anyone too ignorant to get sober. Anyone can be taught. But I've met many people who are too smart to get sober. They try to think their way around the disease and, because of their accomplishments, consider themselves different from the usual stereotypes of the poor, failed, homeless, and sick alcoholic or addict.

In my work, I treat a lot of physicians, and I find them particularly challenging. Why? Many of the qualities that one looks for and admires in physicians work against them in recovery. For example, who wouldn't want a self-sufficient, independent surgeon in absolute control of the operating room during their surgery? If your life were

RAISING THE BAR

A 2016 study conducted by the Hazelden Betty Ford Foundation and the American Bar Association Commission on Lawyer Assistance Programs found that 21 percent of licensed lawyers are problem drinkers. The percentage increases by more than 10 percent for practicing lawyers under the age of 30. Of the more than 19,000 lawyers surveyed, 75 percent skipped over the section on other drug use. Up to 15 percent of health care professionals and less than 1 percent of pilots suffer from alcoholism. The low rate of alcoholism in pilots is most likely due to strict Federal Aviation Administration (FAA) regulations.

at stake, wouldn't you want the ultimate authority and decision maker doing all that is required to get you through an operation? By the same token, who wouldn't want a lawyer who can argue a case against all odds, whose knowledge of the law controls the court room, mesmerizes the jury, and convinces others to think the way he or she is thinking? Who wouldn't want a pilot who, in absolute control, weathers the storm and safely lands passengers on a wet runway on a rainy night?

Those qualities of absolute control, perfectionism, and independent decision making, which work so well in high-stress careers, go against some of the basic principles of recovery. In recovery, mistakes are human. You are asked to give up control, indeed surrender, to a power greater than yourself. Who would choose to leave a world where the power differential was completely in your favor and, if used appropriately, got you exactly what you wanted? The nurse practitioner of an addicted physician may feel absolutely compelled to supply that physician with a prescription, written by her own hand, because her livelihood would be threatened if she didn't agree. In treatment, powerful high achievers are asked to enter a world where the power differential switches, where they must admit powerlessness to the substances that are taking control of their lives. Where they must look at the wreckage of their past and its effect on their family. Where they are patients instead of caregivers, clients rather than attorneys, passengers instead of pilots, subordinates instead of CEOs.

In recovery, high achievers must humbly identify as just another run-of-the-mill alcoholic or addict, one among the 10 percent, at the same level as the butcher, the baker, and the candlestick maker. After years of intense training in their chosen profession, these folks identify with what they do. They are not a father, a husband, or a good man but rather a neurosurgeon, a tax attorney, or a 737 pilot. They identify themselves by their accomplishments and their profession. They have become human doings rather than human beings.

The first target of the disease is awareness, and especially in the case of the professional, the alcoholic or addict is usually the last one to know that he or she has a problem. (If you're reading this and shaking your head, think about why you're reacting this way.) While reading this book is a great first step, a high-functioning addict may require an intervention, either by family or professional committee. Even if the high achiever realizes the truth, he or she may vigorously fight the accusations. This is why the clinical diagnostic evaluation process was invented. This elaborate investigative process uses hair analyses, fingernail analyses, polygraph tests, and testimony from family and work associates to produce overwhelming evidence to convince a person in severe denial that she has a problem—that her current self-perception is distorted and the facts point to inevitable disaster.

If the disease is in question—if the high achiever strongly resists any effort to get help—contacting a residential treatment center to schedule a clinical diagnostic evaluation is the answer. These in-depth evaluations, which sometimes last 3 to 7 days, are becoming more and more common. Via tests, interviews, and observation, a clinical team thoroughly examines the evidence and either confirms or denies that addiction is a problem, could be a problem in the future, or is not a problem.

ENTITLEMENT

Why is it that a high achiever's power to succeed ultimately fails him when attempting to control alcohol or drug use? The answer is tied to feelings and behaviors often learned in adolescence, a time when many of us have some structure that requires our pretense and attention—athletic activities, the yearbook committee, the school newspaper, an after-school job. We learn that we are praised for hard work, and that feels good. We also learn to feel entitled to celebrate on a weekend or a day off. This pattern carries into college, resulting in the binge epidemic we see in colleges today. Students used to drink on Friday and Saturday night. Now oftentimes Thursday night serves as the initiation into the weekend. Students take stimulants such as Ritalin (methylphenidate), prescribed to treat attention-deficit/hyperactivity disorder (ADHD), in an effort to "cure" hangovers so that, on Monday, they can return to classes feeling good.

This pattern, if successful, allows students to party hard and still earn respectable grades. During my first year in medical school, I recall taking an entire 4-day weekend to celebrate after a neuroanatomy examination. My friends and I felt entitled to celebrate the end of an arduous study period with "relaxation behavior" that was way overboard. I upheld this pattern throughout my professional career. I remember walking into a bar and hearing the bartender say, "Gee, Doc, don't you ever stop working? You deserve a drink!" Even my patients were part of my trained sense of entitlement. It worked for about 35 years before the scales were tipped and I was met with irrefutable evidence that I needed help.

Today the use of alcohol among professionals is exposed to far greater scrutiny. Most professional settings have instituted systems for reporting abnormal behaviors, whether it be a hospital well-being committee or an employee-assistance plan. Some states have laws that require physicians to report when a colleague shows up for work impaired. Up to 50 percent of all reports made to hospital well-being committees do not involve cases of suspected chemical impairment but behavioral abnormalities, like inappropriate anger, which are often symptoms of chemical impairment.

However, the belief that one is entitled to binge or abuse alcohol or drugs remains common among highly successful students and professionals. Many are proud of their ability to "work hard, play hard." But this cannot last forever.

TREATMENT

High-functioning addicts are often treated with a period of medically facilitated detoxification and up to 90 days of residential treatment. The treatment team also works to identify any psychological or psychiatric conditions, such as depression, anxiety, bipolar illness, and ADHD, that often coexist with the disease of addiction. These mental health issues may be related to substance abuse and disappear with abstinence, or they may be independent disorders that need to be treated.

Ideal patients enter treatment voluntarily and practice rigorous honesty, a progressive type of honesty that gets better and better as time goes on. They are able to deal with the shame of using substances. They recognize the severity of their illness and are willing to stay in treatment until they are well. They are willing to ask for and accept help. They comply with the rules, accept feedback, and are accountable to other people, including those who have far fewer professional credentials than they do. Many professionals need time to become humble, accept their situation, identify with other people in treatment, and get to the point where they can ask for help and see that their lives have not been working. My experience with professionals is that leverage works: Family, licensure, social position, employment status—if any of these things are hanging in the balance, it gets their attention.

The magic I have seen with people in this group usually happens somewhere between 6 and 8 weeks into treatment. An interesting phenomenon occurs, often described by patients as a period of light, when their resistance drops and they truly identify as an alcoholic or addict. They become more teachable and, at that point, their professional skills and their intelligence become assets to recovery. Now they experience the acceptance and surrender that has eluded them for so long.

It may take high-achieving professionals longer than most other patients, but eventually almost all get into a solid program of recovery. Still, I see no reason to take someone who is new to recovery and bankrupt them. Long-term outpatient concierge treatment is often a viable and more economical alternative to abandoning work and family for months at a time.

During treatment, they learn to listen and identify. They are not the bosses here. They embrace humility and begin to learn the art of rigorous honesty, a practice that slowly deflates the false self-image they and those around them have created. They do this by facing their greatest fear: disclosure.

THE TERROR OF DISCLOSURE

The obstacle to identifying as an alcoholic or addict and accepting recovery is malignant denial. If we're too smart for our own good, we might fail to realize that we've mistakenly defined our sense of personal and family well-being in terms of our professional success.

So we cover up our feelings. Denying feelings and moods is at the heart of the issue of denial. We can deny as much as we like, but it won't necessarily change the way we feel inside. Becoming irritable, resentful, and discontent, we convert those feelings into self-pity, anger, restlessness, and blaming. It's somewhat natural for our brains to want to adjust away from those feelings. If those feelings aren't regularly incurred in the course of our professional life, the feeling of entitlement follows naturally. "Of course I deserve a break. I deserve to relax," we say, in the same way that we deserve a nice toy, a nice home, a great meal, a second bottle of wine.

Disclosing our feelings and who we really are is terrifying at first. After years of training and practice, many addicted professionals have delusions that they have few or no faults. Patients put doctors on a pedestal. High-powered executives manage large staffs that cater to their every need. Students are lauded for getting straight A's. Knowing that it's impossible for any human being to be perfect, these high achievers start to believe they are greater than human. They believe they can control all that is going on around them, including the use of drugs and alcohol. Doctors are particularly susceptible to this thought process. After years of being a healer, the physician believes he can self-diagnose. He is unable to see himself as a patient and cannot find the humility to ask for help. Professional arrogance, the need to be worthy of high expectations and social positions, and the perception that only they and they alone can do their jobs leave high-achieving professionals unable to face the facts.

Treating high-functioning alcoholics or addicts with their peers can be advantageous. Members of these groups are able to call out each other on their BS. They pull the covers back to expose denial for what it is and hold their peers accountable. This honesty has the effect of reducing shame ("I'm not the only one who's taken meds from an elderly patient") and helps break through denial. Patients become more likely to share their consequences in front of a group of people who can't judge them without judging themselves. They begin to take ownership for the consequences they've disconnected from: bankruptcy, health issues, and relationship issues. These professionals, whose self-images and egos are highly organized around their identification with their work, do better when treated together.

My beloved sponsor, Tony T., has a high school education and makes pizzas and is utterly unimpressed with the diplomas on my wall. He sees them, rightly so, as past obstacles to the surrender that was necessary for me to access care.

IN RECOVERY

After treatment, a high-functioning addict must introduce the principles of recovery into his chosen profession, which now takes a backseat to his new primary profession—the work of recovery.

He must pay attention to any signs of cross-addiction, such as nicotine or other drugs, food, sex, or the Internet, which may signal a state of imbalance. We encourage professionals to invest in their recovery just as they have with their education. Recovery capital is deposited on a regular basis. Professionals can look at their recovery as a new form of wealth—one that exists day by day, based upon the work that they put into it and upon their daily spiritual condition.

The true essential of recovery is surrender, which is a new and foreign principle, but one that delivers true fulfillment. Professionals in recovery must completely surrender to their treatment process and long-term recovery. Old resentments and anger must give rise to the spiritual principles of trust and gratitude for the gift of recovery. It is a gift to be cherished. Treatment must be viewed as a positive experience and a measurable marker of sobriety.

THE IMPORTANCE OF MONITORING

In Chapter 9 we'll discuss the issue of relapse and learn some devastating news about its rate of occurrence with the disease of addiction. However, the good news is that professionals such as pilots and physicians have 5-year recovery rates of 78 to 92 percent, well above the average 5-year rate of about 30 percent. How can it be that the most difficult patient is the most compliant once out of treatment? Because physicians, lawyers, and pilots are responsible for the lives of others, they are required by their board or the FAA to be monitored after treatment for 5 years. They sign a contract stating that they can be randomly asked for a urine sample at any time within 5 years after discharge. They agree that they have to prove their sobriety and their active participation in a recovery program, disclosing the meetings that they go to and the counselors they meet.

Ninety-plus percent of professionals in treatment return to work and are gainfully employed. I can't overemphasize the need for monitoring in all strata of patients treated for the disease of addiction. The evidence says it works. This is why we apply the principles of aftercare monitoring to all patients who are treated. The longer the treatment, the longer the monitoring, the better the outcome.

The topic of monitoring takes us back to the high achiever's advanced skill set. This is the stage where the truly smart and manipulative professional can fake it until he makes it and keep on faking it right through the monitoring period after discharge. These people can go for 5 years and pass every drug test, dot every i and cross every t, and at the end of the 5 years they have completed the work and have been absolutely compliant, as a matter of convenience and part of a bargain they made to keep their job or their license.

These folks may have complied, but they never surrendered. Unfortunately, people in this small but significant group fall off the cliff soon after their monitoring contracts end. When they are no longer held accountable, they return to treatment, oftentimes in greater shame and denial than ever before. We approach the relapsing professional in yet a different way, the particulars of which are beyond the scope of this book. Surrender is key and essential to long-term recovery. Otherwise, no matter how long one is monitored, this disease is waiting to resurface.

THE YOUNG PROFESSIONAL

Tom, a young man whom I've known since he was a baby, graduated from an Ivy League school and landed a job with one of the strongest brokerage houses in New York. He became the golden boy, soon acquiring accounts, much to his credit, that left him with great wealth. Within a short time, he bought his first apartment and then his second, which was bigger and better than the first. Like in the movie *Wall Street,* his acquisitions soared. It was not long before his closest friends started saying they thought Tom might be in trouble because he partied a little hard. But to his peers, it looked like more fun than anything: Tom was typically the brunt of well-meaning jokes and the subject in telling photographs on Facebook. He had earned a party reputation, and the number of weekends lost, in fun, to drugs and alcohol started to mount.

During this time, Tom announced that he was getting married. He made it through his entire wedding, though obviously buzzed, without embarrassing himself or his bride, a feat that attested to the enormous tolerance he had acquired for alcohol.

Newly minted professionals often display an acute occurrence of malignant denial in the face of youthful accomplishment. The amount of heartache and ruin, both financial and emotional, to these individuals and their families is too great to measure. The challenge is the notion of invincibility. When young men and women, oftentimes just out of school and holding a new diploma, land a job in a competitive market and start to acquire some of the accoutrements of success—business cards, their own office, a place in the company directory—they begin to feel the power of success.

In their early twenties and on top of the world, they experience wealth and respect, perhaps for the first time, and the stress and pressures that go along with it. These young professionals still don't have a fully developed power of reasoning (the brain's prefrontal cortex continues to develop until age 26). Some young professionals are more likely to use drugs or alcohol with abandon, believing they are not susceptible to harm. How can we intervene before it's too late?

If you're a young professional, how do you know whether your alcohol or drug use is a problem? Start by looking for a state of balance. Are you able to play hard and work hard without tipping the scales toward the point of intoxication, to the point of embarrassment, to the point of slurred speech—all signs that essentially constitute an overdose? That's right: Slurred speech and imbalance signify that the brain is undergoing small amounts of brain damage, disrupting neuropathways and altering brain function.

If you feel out of control, unable to stop even a newly formed habit of drinking after work or getting completely blasted at every company party, it's time to consider getting help. Not only are you damaging your brain cells, you're setting yourself up for a descent into a devastating disease that may ruin all that you are trying to accomplish (not to mention the lives of a spouse and children who may be around the corner).

In recovery we come to understand why it's cool to be sober—it's desirable to have dignity and self-respect. We long for integrity and seek admiration from our colleagues and friends rather than whispers about over-the-top weekend behavior. Maturity replaces invincibility, and we become human. We accept that adulthood brings with it not only wealth and freedom but also responsibility to ourselves, our families, and our employers.

Every time I see a successful intervention on a young person with addiction, I smile with joy, knowing that it represents the rest of his or her life saved.

Don was a graduate of Harvard Medical School and widely published in his chosen medical field. Highly specialized and extraordinarily successful, Don was, most importantly, a terrible alcoholic. Don had been in and out of treatment and felt he knew the ropes. I can remember that day in the detoxification unit, when he looked at me and told me what his diagnosis was. He then told me what his prescription for treatment would be: He would stay no more than 5 to 10 days detoxifying and would then return to his well-worn system back home. He would return to AA and essentially drive his own ship.

Don had self-will like I had never seen before and arrogance beyond the norm. Despite my advice, Don left treatment after 10 days. On his first day at home, Don learned that he might be displaced from his highly regarded and coveted position as a medical director for a very successful firm. Paranoia set in, but he had no sponsor to call and no prime recovery to grasp. He started to ruminate on the idea that he had been rejected, and resentment started to surface. He had visions of an empty office where he had once worked and could even hear an echo. He got the idea that the code on his swipe card had probably been changed. He took his swipe card and went down to the office to see if his office was empty, if he'd been vanquished as a failure. His stress kept mounting. When he got to the office, he found everything as he had left it before he came in for detox, but the anxiety and anticipation were too much for him. He started to drive home but instead pulled into a liquor store, went inside like he had no history at all, grabbed a bottle, and began to drink.

Don returned to us for treatment in far worse condition than before. He was desperate, begging for admission. He looked me in the eyes and said, "My name is Don, and I'm an alcoholic, and, while I am with you, I am not a doctor. I just need help. I'll do anything it takes."

— TAKEAWAYS —

» Addiction doesn't discriminate.

» Staff and family members usually protect the high-achieving addict/alcoholic from being exposed for a lengthy period of time.

» High-achieving professionals, such as doctors, lawyers, and pilots, often benefit from participating in a specialized intensive treatment program with their peers.

» Many of the skills that work for professionals in their careers work against them in recovery.

» Surrender and long-term monitoring are essential for the professional in recovery.

» Overall, high-achieving professionals have a much better success rate in recovery than the general population.

CHAPTER 4

WHAT TO EXPECT
IN RECOVERY

"People who drink to drown their sorrows should be told that sorrow knows how to swim."

—ANN LANDERS

AFTER TREATMENT, I returned to my small town in Vermont and was faced with a very significant dilemma. Because I was required to go to many Twelve Step meetings, I would travel miles and miles, for up to 2 hours, and return home late in the evening after a 1-hour meeting. I remember telling a friend about my new meeting requirements and how difficult it would be to spend so much time on the road away from my family. He said, "Well, Harry, there are probably five or six meetings right here in town. Why don't you try one of them?"

Of course, my answer was simple: "How can I possibly reveal myself to the community, to let them know their doctor is so afflicted with the disease of addiction?"

He smiled. "What's the matter? Are you afraid the rumor will get out that you're getting sober?"

My friend's comment was the defining moment that relieved me of shame. Disclosure was easy, and when I finally walked into that meeting, 3 minutes from my door, right in the middle of town, I ran into a roomful of smiling faces, all saying welcome. One of those smiling faces, patting an empty chair, said, "We've been saving this one for you, Doc."

We keep talking about recovery, but what exactly is it? Ultimately, recovery is living a full and meaningful life without relying on drugs or alcohol. Recovery is a safe place where we explore new ground, where we can open up our gifts, talents, and creativity and share them with the world. In recovery, we have a love of life and are able to have just plain fun.

Like the disease of addiction, recovery is also progressive. At first, we learn not to fear the water, and then we learn how to swim. We move on to snorkeling, and we see below the surface. Then we get our oxygen tanks, dive deep, and discover that underneath there exists a whole new world we never before imagined, and it keeps getting better and better and better.

Recovery takes time and effort. Is it worth all the effort? In rehabilitation with a broken leg, we hope to gain back 80 or 90 percent of our original function. Rarely do we approach or get back to 100 percent. In recovery from addiction, however, we get back much more than we ever had before, even at the top of our game while we were using: 150 to 200 percent and more is an achievable goal.

So, yes, it's worth it. But experience shows us that recovery doesn't happen overnight. Recovery happens in stages and involves a few big learning curves. So you understand what you're getting into, let's break recovery down into three stages:

1. We learn how to stop using alcohol and other drugs.
2. We learn how to cope without using alcohol and other drugs.
3. We learn how to live a full life without using alcohol and other drugs.

Let's take a closer look at each stage of recovery.

HOW TO STOP

As I explained in Chapter 1, our body chemistry won't allow us to continue using drugs without losing control. Once an addict, always an addict. Once addicted, always addicted. We are never "recovered" but always "in recovery." We are never cured; we are always a work in progress.

Abstinence

If we have the disease of addiction, we need to lower the dopamine bell, and the only way to do that is to abstain from using chemicals. This means all mood-altering chemicals and behaviors. We must create an environment where our brains can begin to heal and regain full function. We take it one day at a time—we will not drink or use for this day. If we can't imagine making it through the day without a drink/hit/snort, we can at first try it for an hour at a time.

Abstinence is easier if we realize that our drug or alcohol use has created some cognitive damage. In other words, mentally, we aren't functioning at peak performance, and some of us may be one sandwich shy of a picnic for the time being. Our brains won't heal until we abstain for a period of time, and abstaining is harder when we can't think clearly. But the good news is that, over a period of a few weeks, our brain realizes that the flow of dopamine has stopped. Our brain responds by lowering the dopamine bell, increasing the number of dopamine receptors, and revving up its own dopamine-producing engines. And we start to feel better. We start to feel good without the aid of drugs or alcohol.

But be aware that the brain remembers. If we start using again, our dopamine bell returns to its highest height. It may take a minute or it may take a few weeks or months, but our dopamine bell will go back to where it was when we were using the most. The result is an uncontrollable craving for drugs or alcohol, and we're right back where we started. When we accept this scientifically proven fact, we accept the need for abstinence from drugs and alcohol.

The common obsession of every alcoholic and addict is the idea that we'll be able to use normally. This never happens. This is the essence of the realization of our powerlessness, of our hijacked brain. In recovery, we accept the fact that once a pickle, we cannot go back to being a cucumber. From here, we start learning how to cope without chemicals.

Cycling

Cycling is going through periods of abstinence followed by relapse, or returning to drugs or alcohol. Many of us cycle for years. At some point early on we know we're alcoholics or addicts and that we need

ABSTINENCE VERSUS "HARM REDUCTION"

I've met many people who were not ready to give up every drug. They wanted to continue smoking marijuana or could give up alcohol but not the Xanax (alprazolam), or could stop taking the opioids but still needed to take something for their anxiety. Many of these folks try programs that don't require total and complete abstinence.

There are many, many roads to recovery, and I never knock any of them. In my experience, programs that do not promote complete abstinence wind up allowing the participant to use other substances, and they are soon back on the drug of choice or something similar and in as much trouble as they were before. I'm all for harm reduction—for backing off, for reducing use—but eventually, if you want the recovery I talk about in this book, abstinence from mood-altering chemicals is the mainstay. It is what we shoot for.

help, but we postpone getting it, sometimes for decades. We enter into periods of abstinence, and then we struggle and quickly relapse. Some of us never have a real recovery to relapse from. There's a belief system that allows us to continue the cycle over and over again, and it's based on a false sense of security. The cycling is our disease disguising itself and progressing. The disease says, "You deserve to be able to drink or use normally." Then the disease comes back and uses our weakness against us.

One of the surest ways of continuing the cycle of addiction is to identify only a single substance as the problem. Some of us are on what I call the marijuana maintenance program. That's when we abstain from alcohol completely, attend Alcoholics Anonymous meetings, and kind of keep quiet the fact that once or twice a week we

still smoke a joint. It is only a matter of time before the opportunity
to drink alcohol comes up while we're under the influence of marijuana. Our guard is down, our inhibitions are down, and it isn't long
before we give ourselves permission because we really deserve to have
a drink, and then another. And the cycle starts all over again. This
happens frequently with those of us who stay on diet pills, pain pills,
or sleep medications. I can truthfully say that I had 2-, 3-, and 5-year
periods during which I did not drink alcohol but was not abstinent
from all mood-altering chemicals. During those years, and under the
right conditions, the cycle was easily restarted.

Detox and Withdrawal Symptoms

When I was physician director at the Betty Ford Center, we asked
new patients to arrive at our doorstep under the influence (provided
they were not driving themselves, of course). Yes, we wanted them to
come to us drunk or high.

Why would we encourage patients to do this? It wasn't so they
could have one last hurrah. Primarily, it was a safety measure. We
didn't want patients to start detoxing before treatment. For many,
especially alcoholics, detoxification is dangerous and deadly and
should be medically supervised.

Detoxification is the process of clearing the drugs or alcohol from
the body, and in some people this creates intense withdrawal symptoms. Most people experience at least some major or minor discomfort
for several days. For the heavy drinker, detox can bring convulsions,
hallucinations, delirium tremens (known as the D.T.'s), anxiety, shaki-
ness, heart attack, and even death. Heroin addicts feel physical pain
for the first time since they started using. Cocaine addicts experience
insomnia, anxiety, and depression. Everyone experiences cravings.

A medically supervised detox can alleviate withdrawal symptoms when they are at their worst and most dangerous.

Addiction professionals do not take the life-threatening process of detoxification lightly, and there is absolutely no need to suffer through it without help. With the medications we have now, and given time and the proper setting, we can safely bring a patient off even the most dangerous drug combinations at high doses. Just as we wouldn't put a scalpel in the hands of an amateur surgeon, we should not try to manage detoxification on our own.

My point is: Do not do this at home. Seek help from a competent, medically supervised detoxification program, such as those found at a local hospital or treatment center. They are available at most hospitals, and they are not terribly expensive. Most health insurance policies cover detox, and many county programs offer medically supervised detox at a minimal cost.

The old cold turkey scenario is simply no longer necessary. Make sure you use a properly supervised medical detox program. Do not do this on your own.

Cravings

Once we're beyond detox, cravings are probably one of the most bothersome withdrawal symptoms. The worst of the cravings happens during detox, when the body is shocked by the sudden absence of the drug it has come to know and love. But cravings for our drug of choice can linger sometimes for days, weeks, months, or, in rare cases, even years. And cravings can return. We can be carefree, whistling a tune while we walk down the street, only to pass a bar and catch a whiff of a familiar scent. Boom, we crave a beer or a shot of whiskey. But cravings do diminish. They get weaker, shorter, and further and further apart. The important thing in early recovery is to have a plan for what to do when a craving strikes (and it will strike).

Here are some ideas:

Make a list of 10, 20, or 30 things you could do other than drink or use. Keep the list close by and update it when you come up with new ideas. I'm talking about fun, creative things that will enhance your life and the lives of others. (Your recovery is not just about you!)

Use your energy productively by working out or walking around the block. You need to use your body; it will respond in a dramatic way. You owe it to your body, especially if you have been abusing it for a long time.

Remember why you're in recovery now. What consequences got you here? Don't just remember the good times you had. Play the tape in your head through to the end and recall that you almost lost your children/ your spouse/your job/your dignity/your life. This is called keeping it green. Never forget. Try not to remember your last drink, but always remember your last drunk. We want to make sure that we remember where drugs and alcohol take us—the loss of control. Don't call it a buzz if it was really an overdose.

Call someone you trust and talk through your craving. Tell him or her what you're feeling. Talking about it has the remarkable effect of diminishing its power over us. It's truly amazing.

Know that most cravings only last 30 seconds. Identify it, talk about it, and put it out there. You can even keep a material object, like a doll or some other totem, nearby. When a craving comes, look at it, talk to it, whack it with the back of your hand, and move it out of your life.

Sit with the craving. Don't fight it, but close your eyes, allow yourself to feel it wash over you, and then let it go.

Change your self-talk. Inside, you might be screaming, *I need a drink!* Consider whose voice that is for a minute and then take over. You can just as easily say, *I want a drink, but I don't need one right now. I'll do . . . for the next 2 minutes and see how I'm feeling then.* Set a timer if you'd like. Meanwhile, play the tape in your head: *If I do have the drink that I think I want, it will turn into 5, 6, or 10 drinks. I will then get drunk, embarrass myself, hurt myself and others, fall down the stairs, get arrested, go to the emergency room, and awaken the dragon that will distort my life and the lives of those around me.* Might as well call a spade a spade.

Avoid going to slippery places. Slippery places include bars, parties, and neighborhoods where drugs are sold. It's important to stay away from these places, especially in early recovery. If you can't miss a major family event, such as your sister's wedding, make sure to plan ahead. Bookend the event with calls to a sponsor (or bring your sponsor along) and have your own transportation so you can leave early if necessary.

HOW TO COPE

Despite our body's natural ability to heal itself, like many inheritable diseases, addiction is a tough disease to tackle. Abstinence, detox, and dealing with cravings are a huge part of recovery. But abstinence alone will not cure what ails us. Abstinence is just the beginning. We're required to do a lot more.

The good news is there's help to get us through the upcoming stages. There's a tried-and-true plan that has worked for millions of others in your situation. You've most likely heard of the Twelve Steps. Someone close to you may have told you to go to Alcoholics Anonymous (AA) or Narcotics Anonymous (NA) meetings. Most likely, you resisted. "I don't need AA. I can quit on my own anytime. I don't go to groups. I'm not interested in wasting my time hanging out with a bunch of people telling old stories over and over again. I know I can quit. I've done it many times."

Yes, anyone can quit, but we need to be able to quit *for good*. That requires that we surrender to this disease and have a plan in place to help us cope, without drugs or alcohol, through good times and bad times.

As a recovering alcoholic and as director of a concierge treatment program, I see people just like you every day. While your situation, your personality, your biology, and your history are unique to you, addictive behavior and its consequences are predictable. And to a certain degree, so is the path you take to find peace and serenity. Twelve Step-based programs have helped millions of people to recover from addiction and lead fulfilling, productive lives. We start by using the Twelve Steps to learn how to cope with whatever stress life throws at us—difficult relationships, pressure at work, loss, success—without going back to our chemicals.

HOW TO LIVE

At first we use the Twelve Step program of recovery to cope with our discomfort, physical and emotional, as a clean and sober person. Before we know it, we are using the Twelve Steps as a guide for how to live: Our coping is transformed into living. We no longer fear adversity, but we welcome it as an opportunity to use our newly acquired principles, discipline, and skills, such as absolute rigorous honesty and courage to take action with integrity. Through the Twelve Steps, we have a belief system that resonates with us, and we act accordingly.

In each day and each moment, we anticipate the joys and are no longer concerned with the fears of the inevitable. We do not fear death. We are prepared. We challenge our resentments, enjoy our human-ness, and are always becoming a better man/woman, husband/wife, father/mother, brother/sister, boss/employee, with gratitude and humility. We keep this new life not by holding on to it but by sharing it with others at every opportunity.

— TAKEAWAYS —

» Recovery is leading a full and meaningful life without relying on drugs or alcohol.

» Like addiction, recovery is progressive.

» For our brains to heal, abstinence is required.

» A medically supervised detoxification is always recommended. For some people, an unsupervised detox can be lethal.

» Cravings diminish over time but can strike at any time.

» We can use many different methods to deal with cravings, including distraction and letting go.

» The Twelve Step program outlines everything we need to cope in life without our drug of choice.

» Before we know it, the Twelve Steps become a cherished way of life.

CHAPTER 5

THE TWELVE STEPS: AS SIMPLE AS IT GETS

"Just 'cause you got the monkey off your back doesn't mean the circus has left town."

—George Carlin

ADDICTION SPECIALISTS CALL it rock bottom. I refer to it as the year from hell.

In a short span of time, I lost a small medical practice and a large investment in California; lost my mother to a prolonged illness; was arrested and charged with a DUI (during the same period of time I was testifying in court on behalf of a patient charged with a DUI); declared bankruptcy; and underwent surgery to remove a portion of my colon, which meant I was now forced to excrete bowel movements using a colostomy bag.

When I was back on my feet physically but still in denial about the severity of my addiction, I decided on a 30-day sabbatical to "take the cure." *Piece of cake*, I thought. Ten days of Ayurvedic healing at a spa in southern Colorado, 10 days of skiing in Steamboat Springs—where there is a martini named for me—and then I would finish up at some place called the Betty Ford Center for their 10-day program.

Robert Millman, a friend and well-known addiction expert from New York, made the arrangements. "I was just at the Betty Ford Center," he said. "They have this great program for professionals, and it's only 10 days. You're going to love it."

On March 1, I arrived at the Betty Ford Center and told them I was there for the 10-day program. They laughed and said they had no 10-day program. Their program for licensed health care professionals was 90 days minimum. Surprise!

I hemmed and hawed and said they couldn't possibly get me for that long. I had people back home who depended on me. In retrospect, they also depended on me to be sober—a thought that eluded me at the time.

I was there when they spoke to Cheryl, my office manager, who said, "Keep him. He's broken. Don't send him back until he's fixed."

I was paranoid that my medical records and treatment for this disease would become known, so I used an alias and my brother Tom's date of birth during admission. Because I was still shrouded in shame and denial, my acceptance and surrender weren't going to come easy.

Before the luggage search, I did what any other alcoholic or drug addict would do before entering treatment for 3 months. I opened my shaving kit, threw away the batteries from my flashlight, and replaced them with as much speed (in the form of a diet pill I took to keep me alert) as I could cram into the compartment. It would only hold 68 hits, so I wound up staring at what remained—20 mostly broken and crumbled pieces in the cup of my hand. What would you do if you looked in your hand and saw that? I swallowed them, of course. So I was awake and alert long enough to read the Big Book eight times. By 4:00 a.m., I opened up the flashlight and threw its contents into the toilet, watching as the last piece with the little blue specks began to bleach out and blend into the water. Not quite ready to give it up, I quickly reached down and grabbed it. Then I finally let it go and watched it swirl its way into oblivion. I finally had a sobriety date.

To this day, my friend Bob Newton has a cartoon up on the wall back in his counseling room. It is signed by "Harry Louis," the alias I used when admitting myself to the Betty Ford Center years ago, a reminder of the place where I made progress, one day at a time.

I frequently give a lecture on the medical consequences of the disease of addiction. During this lecture, I show extremely graphic photographs of various organ systems of the human body that are most severely affected by alcohol and other drugs. The audience gasps as I move from slide to slide. The brain scans are frightening: Long-term drug use literally creates holes in the brain's tissue. The consequences of the disease of addiction are not just biological; the toll is also psychological, social, and spiritual. But we must recover physically first so that we can grasp the bigger components of recovery.

THE CHALLENGE

Cognitive deficit, or trouble remembering and thinking clearly, is demonstrated in a large percentage of new admissions to alcohol and drug treatment. Measurable by sophisticated testing, affected brain functions include, but are not limited to, cognition, thought, memory, and problem solving. They present the addict or alcoholic with a significant challenge: In the early stages of recovery, we are removed from our best friend, our prime coping mechanism—our drug of choice—and we're told it is time to solve the inevitable problems of life, to take life on life's terms. And we have to contemplate all of this using a damaged brain.

Trying to access the tools of recovery, learn the system, and put it into practice with an impaired brain is in itself quite stressful. The good news is that for most people the damage is temporary, and a remarkable recovery is possible, especially after a period of abstinence.

GETTING THE TWELVE STEP MESSAGE IN EARLY RECOVERY

The brain is a most remarkable organ in its ability to regain lost ground. After several weeks of abstinence, the brain's problem-solving ability, processing speed, and memory show demonstrable improvement. But by that time, many residential patients are already packing their bags and getting ready to step out into the world as a sober man or woman, perhaps for the first time in years. The Twelve Step message escapes many people in early recovery, and it's not because they are stupid. In fact, some studies correlate addiction with above average intelligence. Addicts in early recovery are cognitively impaired, working with a brain damaged by drugs and alcohol. Yet getting the Twelve Step message is imperative to recovery. It's the link between abstinence and recovery. The Steps teach us how to get out of our own way. They get us to understand there's no way we can stay in this fight and win. We see that others have used the Twelve Step method to stop the insanity and realize that we can, too, if we take the same well-worn steps.

In a 28-day inpatient treatment program, patients are expected to get through the first five of the Twelve Steps. That may not sound like much, but it's a lot when you consider learning a new emotionally and spiritually based language while suffering from impaired thinking. Many patients struggle. Unless newcomers stick with it after treatment by attending AA or NA meetings and keeping the faith that the Twelve Step message will click someday, the temptation to start drinking or using is high.

A Very Simple Concept

In my experience, the cognitive difficulties we have when entering a treatment program and being introduced to the Twelve Steps prevent us from understanding a very simple concept. And although I have never seen anyone too stupid or too cognitively disrupted or impaired to get this simple program eventually, I have seen many people too smart to get it. How so? The Steps may not be too difficult to understand intellectually, but to embrace them emotionally, engage with them, and take action because of them is the real challenge for many people. To the newcomer, the Twelve Steps and the principles they embrace seem to be written in a foreign language.

THE BIG BOOK

The Big Book is how most people refer to *Alcoholics Anonymous*, a book first published in 1939 and currently in its fourth edition. The book got its nickname because of the thick paper used in the first printing to bulk up the book and, hence, the perceived value. The Big Book is considered by many to be one of the most influential books of all time, spearheading Twelve Step recovery—one of the largest social movements of the 20th century. To date, the Big Book has been translated into more than 50 languages and has sold about 35 million copies.

THE BACKBONE OF THE TWELVE STEP PROGRAM

Because understanding the Twelve Steps is crucial to recovery, and cognitive deficits in early recovery can make understanding the Twelve Steps difficult, let's review the basic tenets of the program. Then I'll present a simple version—my version of the Twelve Steps.

One Step at a Time

The Twelve Steps are suggestions only. Importantly, it is suggested that we take them one at a time and in order, each being built upon the foundation of the previous step. Step Four, for instance, asks us to take an inventory of our lives that is searching and fearless. We cannot accomplish this until we get through Step Three, where we abandon that fear by turning it over to our Higher Power or, as the Steps word it, to "God as we understand Him."

Spiritual versus Religious Program

The Twelve Steps were never meant to be a religious program but one of a spiritual nature. It's important to note that, in the Steps, the concept of God has a wide range of meanings and can embrace any number of people and their cultures and histories. We are free to replace the term *God* with any power greater than ourselves: spiritual enlightenment, Higher Power, even our Twelve Step group. What's important is that we acknowledge that there is a power greater than ourselves.

The Steps help us to achieve wholeness, or integrity, between our belief systems (our inner self) and our actions (our outer self). Here we form a cohesive life in harmony with our deepest values. We see how we've acted against our values and learn to live so that our actions and beliefs walk together, hand in hand. We finally decide to do the right thing.

Lessons in How to Live Life

The Steps are really about living life. Alcohol is only mentioned once (in the First Step). The number of Twelve Step meetings dealing with different problems has mushroomed over the years, so that alcohol is replaced with gambling, codependency, sex addiction, food addiction, cocaine, or some other addiction. The common denominator is that all participants are looking to recover and live a meaningful life, and that is the essence of the Twelve Steps.

Powerful Language

The Twelve Steps use some powerful terms: defects, wrongs, and shortcomings. The language is not meant to make us feel bad about ourselves but to get us to confront our self-righteous pride. The language is strong, but when we are rigorously honest with ourselves and others, we realize that the word choices are spot on. And instead of feeling bad, we feel a freedom we've never known. Worded as they are, the Steps hold us accountable for our behaviors, past and present, and create a safe place for us to begin the work of recovery.

Only You Alone Can Do It, but You Cannot Do It Alone

Although we may spend time alone with our thoughts and in meditation or prayer, recovery doesn't take place in isolation. It happens in the Twelve Step Fellowship, a wonderfully supportive group of men and women who share their experiences, hopes, and strengths with each other, helping to cultivate gratitude. Through the Fellowship, we know we are not alone, and we realize how much our recovery depends on participating and serving.

DR. HARRY'S TWELVE STEPS

When I was in early recovery, I took the liberty of rewording the Steps so I could better grasp their meaning. These somewhat comical but honest interpretations have helped provide enormous clarity for me and for many of my patients in getting started on the road to a new life. Notice that each step includes a one-word principle, or a spiritual code of conduct, along with its opposite—a character defect. We can look at each spiritual principle as the gift we get from working through each particular step.

— Step One —

ORIGINAL:

We admitted we were powerless over alcohol—that our lives had become unmanageable.

TRANSLATION:

There is a power that wants to kill me.

CHARACTER DEFECT:

Denial

SPIRITUAL PRINCIPLE:

Honesty

Now that translation touches my soul enough to scare me. My addiction is active, relentless, going after my family and all aspects of my life, health, finances, and relationship with God. This step confronts denial and brings awareness of the unmanageability of our lives into focus. Here we accept our identity as alcoholics or addicts. We accept that our Higher Power has been our drug of choice. The principle of this step is the foundation for all other work: *absolute rigorous honesty.* The character defects it confronts are dishonesty and denial, the prime tools alcoholics and addicts use to continue in their destructive lifestyles. If we accept our identity as an alcoholic or addict, we finally realize that only through rigorous honesty can we see the consequences of our continued use and take responsibility. We understand that powerlessness means that we cannot attempt to control our drug of choice. Use of our will is only met with greater consequences.

— Step Two —

ORIGINAL:

Came to believe that a Power greater than ourselves could restore us to sanity.

TRANSLATION:

There is a power that wants me to live.

CHARACTER DEFECT:

Despair

SPIRITUAL PRINCIPLE:

Hope

What a concept! Here we're confronted with the notion that continuing to use or drink despite the fact that we're sitting on a pile of adverse consequences (DUIs, divorce, debt, job loss) is insane. It's insane to think that someday we will be able to use normally. The sane thing to do is to fire the old Higher Power (drugs and alcohol) and find a more promising Higher Power—one that's on our side. The principle here is hope; the character defect, despair, which brings into focus the spiritual aspect of this disease. *Why me, God? Perhaps my family would be better off without me. Is there no way out?* Step Two answers that: Yes, there is a way out.

—— Step Three ——

ORIGINAL:

Made a decision to turn our will and our lives over to the care of God *as we understood Him.*

TRANSLATION:

Do I want to live or die?

CHARACTER DEFECT:

Self-will

SPIRITUAL PRINCIPLES:

Faith and surrender

We've now seen that there is a power that wants to kill us and there is a power that wants us to live. Are we willing to give up control and turn our will over to a Higher Power outside of ourselves (the power that wants us to live)? That would seem to be the wisest decision. And in this step, that's all we do—decide to live. Many people turn back at this point, but if we get through Step Three, the rewards are numerous. The principles are faith and surrender, based on the hope attained in Step Two. The third step confronts doubt. Our will is trying to control drinking or drugging. We are obsessed with the notion that we can control addiction and blinded by the evidence to the contrary (our negative consequences, such as loss of family, friends, or job). Our will gets us to this place. The will of our designated Higher Power is, among other things, for us to be good, loving, and sober human beings.

Steps One through Three deal with recognizing that there is a problem *and* a solution. The problem is not only physical and psychological but also spiritual. The solution, therefore, must also be spiritual. The purpose of these first few steps is to establish a relationship based on trust and hope with a power greater than ourselves. It calls upon us to recognize that we must take specific actions, in the steps that follow, to keep and maintain the gift, or the solution to our problem.

—— Step Four ——

ORIGINAL:

Made a searching and fearless moral inventory of ourselves.

TRANSLATION:

Using examples from your life, understand that your actions were controlled by selfishness, dishonesty, fear, and resentment.

CHARACTER DEFECT:

Fear

SPIRITUAL PRINCIPLE:

Courage

A searching and fearless moral inventory is a written list of our dominant character traits. Character traits can be positive or negative: pride, selfishness, compassion. They drive our thinking and behavior whether we're aware of them or not. Our negative character traits, or flaws, separate us from our Higher Power, and they prevent us from connecting with others and experiencing life fully. Completing this inventory is not only vital to our recovery but also an important education. We learn much about ourselves and our perspectives—so much so that we might, for instance, find that none of the resentments we harbor has reason to exist.

TOP 20 CHARACTER DEFECTS

To complete Step Four, we need to put pen to paper. In this exercise, the most important thing is to be honest. Ask yourself how each of the defects below has manifested itself in your life and then write down your answers. You don't need to beat yourself up. This exercise is just meant to help you see your beliefs and behavior more clearly.

1. Resentment, anger
2. Fear, cowardice
3. Self-pity
4. Self-justification
5. Self-importance, egotism
6. Self-condemnation, guilt
7. Lying, evasiveness, dishonesty
8. Impatience
9. Hate
10. False pride, phoniness, denial
11. Jealousy
12. Envy
13. Laziness
14. Procrastination
15. Insincerity
16. Negative thinking
17. Immoral thinking
18. Perfectionism, intolerance
19. Criticizing, loose talk, gossip
20. Greed

Our inventory must be based on faith and trust and approached without fear—that is, with complete honesty. Steps Two and Three have given us faith and trust. Step Four embraces the principle of courage and confronts the defect of fear. Here we do some serious soul searching.

A moral inventory does not just list liabilities; it lists assets as well. We are never all bad, and it's appropriate to recognize our good traits. And the defects of character listed for each step do not necessarily mean the presence of something bad in one's life. A defect may simply mean the absence of something good, such as not enough love, concern, compassion, or consideration or the absence of faith and trust. I'll also add awareness and acceptance to that list. In Step Four, we identify what it is exactly that makes up all the deadweight we're carrying around.

There are several ways to approach a Step Four inventory, and all involve time and effort. We are required to think about past and current life events and then put pen to paper. The following exercise is a good start to help you identify your behavior. There are also workbooks and online resources available, or you can talk to others in recovery for advice. *Alcoholics Anonymous* (the Big Book) also offers an outline on how to do a Step Four inventory.

Resentment: The Biggest Roadblock

The most dominant character defect of alcoholics and addicts tends to be resentment. Resentment goes hand in hand with other character defects, including fear, selfishness, dishonesty, and being inconsiderate. Doing this exercise can help you quickly identify a lot of deadweight in your life.

Use the prompts below to fill in the Step Four Inventory Chart on the following page. Fill in the chart column by column. In other words, finish the first column before moving on to the second and so forth.

First, list every resentment you can think of. List every person, institution, principle, rule, or law that has upset you. This may take a while and turn into a very long list. That's okay. Just be thorough and fearless when making your list.

Next, indicate why you are resentful. What did he/she/it do? What was the result? When you're finished, read this column over. What stands out? Are you mad at he/she/it or at what he/she/it *did* or *represents?* Would you be just as upset if another person, place, or thing made the same offense?

Write down how this affected you. Following is a list from the Big Book of the most common ways our resentments interfere with our sense of self. They are: (1) self-esteem, (2) pride, (3) personal relationships, (4) material security, (5) emotional security, (6) acceptable sexual relations (not hidden), (7) hidden sexual relations, and (8) ambitions.

What was our role? The last question is important. Here we look at each resentment, forgetting about everyone and everything else, and consider our role. What did we do to help cause the situation or make it worse? Were we selfish, dishonest, fearful, and/or inconsiderate?

This exercise helps us to see that we are not always the victims. Sometimes, we play a role in the negative events in our lives. The good news is that, if we play a role in our own resentment, we can forgive ourselves and move on. We no longer give the control, the power over the situation, to the person, place, or thing we are resentful toward. To relieve our burden, he/she/it doesn't have to change; we do.

If it helps, you can use this chart for each character defect you've identified.

STEP FOUR INVENTORY CHART

Character Defect: _____

I RESENT: _____

_____

_____

_____

BECAUSE HE/SHE/IT CAUSED: _____

_____

_____

_____

AND THIS AFFECTS MY: _____

_____

_____

_____

HOW DID I CONTRIBUTE? (SELFISH, DISHONEST, FEARFUL, INCONSIDERATE)

_____

_____

_____

_____

— Step Five —

ORIGINAL:

Admitted to God, to ourselves, and to another human being the exact nature of our wrongs.

TRANSLATION:

Tell your entire embarrassing story to someone in a safe, nonjudgmental setting.

CHARACTER DEFECT:

Dishonesty

SPIRITUAL PRINCIPLE:

Integrity

In Step Five, we bring the inventory we made in Step Four to light. We expose it (and ourselves) to our Higher Power and to another trustworthy individual, such as a sponsor, a spiritual counselor, or a clergyman or woman. This exercise was first recorded in 1935 by Alcoholics Anonymous founders Bill W. and Dr. Bob. In a safe environment, the two men were able to hear and identify with each other's stories and in doing so were released of their burdens. Admitting the exact nature of our wrongs (telling someone our character defects) diminishes the power they have over us. In telling our stories, we expose our shame. We see our acts for what they are. We are no longer shameful or fearful. We are relieved of our past burdens.

In Step Five, we develop honesty and relieve anxiety as we embrace the principle of truth, which becomes our gateway to integrity. When we have integrity, we adhere to a code of values—we are incorruptible. Acting with integrity puts us in a state of completeness. We are undivided; we are whole. I know of no other principle that warms the heart of the alcoholic or addict more than when first touched by integrity. Its absence in one's life is palpable, and when an individual in recovery starts to reclaim it, there is a glow like no other in his eyes. This Twelve Step magic is repeated time and time again.

— Step Six —

ORIGINAL:

Were entirely ready to have God remove all these defects of character.

REVISION:

Decide whether we want to live this way anymore.

CHARACTER DEFECT:

Stubbornness

SPIRITUAL PRINCIPLE:

Willingness

In Step Four, we identified our defects of character. In Step Five, we exposed them. In Step Six, we are simply ready and willing to have our Higher Power remove the defects of character for us. What a gift. Here we decide we no longer want to be dishonest, selfish, greedy, controlling, or whatever defects we claim. All we need here is a willingness to allow this new power into our lives on a daily basis to remove the defects of character that have wreaked such havoc in our lives. Sometimes we start a journey just by being willing to take the first baby step.

— Step Seven —

ORIGINAL:

Humbly asked Him to remove our shortcomings.

TRANSLATION:

If you want to change, ask for help.

CHARACTER DEFECT:

Pride

SPIRITUAL PRINCIPLE:

Humility

It takes us Steps Four, Five, and Six to get to the point where we are ready to ask our Higher Power to remove our character defects, and here we are. Many of us take Step Seven on our knees as we embrace the principle of humility, the essential principle without which no alcoholic or addict can ever recover. This exercise demonstrates humility and the alcoholic's ability, no matter how big the ego, to get down to the level of any other alcoholic or addict, to dare to be average and humbly identify with his or her suffering or pain. This step has been credited as a working principle of Twelve Step recovery. If we want to change, we ask for help and recognize that help and a partnership are prerequisites for change. All kinds of antisocial behaviors disappear when we confront self-righteous pride.

—— Step Eight ——

ORIGINAL:

Made a list of all persons we had harmed and became willing to make amends to them all.

TRANSLATION:

Figure out how to make all our wrongs right.

CHARACTER DEFECT:

Self-centeredness

SPIRITUAL PRINCIPLE:

Reflection and brotherly love

With this list, we need to be thorough and look at relationships that may have started many years ago but still come up as unfinished business. If they require space in our head, they qualify for a place on the list. This list includes people we have hurt, stolen from, betrayed. And it almost always includes people we resented. If we did the resentment exercise in Step Four and finished the fourth section, we know that we were unable to own our part, the role we played, in our resentments. We were self-centered, and so we divested ourselves of responsibility and unfairly blamed the person we resented. This is especially true for those who may have tried to make us aware of what we were doing, only to meet our wrath and mortification. As a result, we harmed the people we resented.

Step Eight is where brotherly love confronts resentment. Resentment is the acid that consumes the vessel that contains it. It has consumed alcoholics and addicts in the past and prevented their recovery.

Until resentment is confronted and resolved, we have little hope of moving on. In Step Eight, we make our list and, using our sponsor or counselor as a guide, we pray for the people we have harmed.

—— Step Nine ——

ORIGINAL:

Made direct amends to such people wherever possible, except when to do so would injure them or others.

TRANSLATION:

Fix what we can without causing more trouble.

CHARACTER DEFECT:

Unfairness and resentment

SPIRITUAL PRINCIPLE:

Justice

We make efforts to repair the damage we created in our past. Making amends means making a change, not just saying "I'm sorry" again. It is the essential healing mechanism of the Twelve Steps that restores relationships with the principles of justice and fairness. Step Nine requires us to be fearless. We make amends even if we are embarrassed or afraid. When we cannot make amends—either because it would cause more harm, because the person is deceased, or because we cannot locate the person—we remain willing (Step Eight) to make amends and do so in our prayers.

Making amends is a cleansing. Once we are cleansed, we do our daily maintenance. We repeat Steps Eight and Nine daily. Every day, we must keep up with the emotional debts that we accumulate. In doing so, we keep our slate clean. We prohibit resentment from creeping into our lives again. We maintain the integrity we've worked so hard to own.

— Step Ten —

ORIGINAL:

Continued to take personal inventory, and when we were wrong, promptly admitted it.

TRANSLATION:

Mistakes are human.

CHARACTER DEFECT:

Procrastination

SPIRITUAL PRINCIPLE:

Vigilance and perseverance

Mistakes happen when we try to live life on life's terms, but we must stay current with these mistakes. Here we bundle up Steps Four through Nine in an effort to keep our slate clean moving forward. If we take a daily inventory and make amends on a daily basis, we will not accumulate these negative influences in our lives. When someone comes to us and says, "I'm so sorry that I did this or that, or that I hurt your feelings or walked right over you," we remember. This display of honesty is a meaningful and powerful episode. We're likely to admire, and might even be inspired to model, this person.

In Step Ten, we assume responsibility for the consequences with those we love. The principle here is perseverance. The character defect is procrastination. For our vigilance, we are rewarded with full and meaningful relationships.

— Step Eleven —

ORIGINAL:

Sought through prayer and meditation to improve our conscious contact with God *as we understood Him,* praying only for knowledge of His will for us and the power to carry that out.

TRANSLATION:

Ask our Higher Power for help in treating others as we would want to be treated by our Higher Power.

CHARACTER DEFECT:

Aimlessness

SPIRITUAL PRINCIPLE:

Awareness

Sounds like the Golden Rule to me. This is not new. The Twelve Steps are not new. These principles have been around for ages. In Step Eleven, we spend more time praying and meditating. We make a conscious effort to connect with our Higher Power throughout the day. We don't stop with one prayer. We talk to and consult our Higher Power throughout the day. Through this communion, we enhance our spiritual power. We naturally improve our relationship with self and others. Our tolerance toward others grows, and we take responsibility for ourselves. This is the essence of spiritual awareness that is missing in the alcoholic or addict who is still using, and it is absolutely essential in the recovery process. The aimlessness stops, and there is a new direction, one that allows us to truly care for others and reap the spiritual benefits in our own lives.

—— Step Twelve ——

ORIGINAL:

Having had a spiritual awakening as the result of these steps, we tried to carry this message to alcoholics and to practice these principles in all our affairs.

TRANSLATION:

Pass it on.

CHARACTER DEFECT:

Selfishness

SPIRITUAL PRINCIPLE:

Service and charity

We practice the principles of Steps One through Eleven, and now with the principles of service and charity, we can pass the program and its principles along to others in need, the way it was given to us. Sharing, not preaching, brings freedom from self-centeredness, and recovery is our new spiritual focus. It is said that to keep it, we need to give it away. Once we are in Step Twelve, we have a spiritual need to give back. If we want to keep the joy of recovery, we need to help others find it. When we serve, we might make coffee at a Twelve Step meeting or help a family intervene with their addicted loved one in a time of crisis. All service has purpose and meaning.

THERE FOR THE TAKING

The Twelve Steps are grace itself—that unconditional gift of love from a Higher Power whose will is to see us healthy and sober. I've written this chapter to explain each step in terms that might be more understandable for those of us knocking at the door of recovery. Before judging the appropriateness of the Twelve Step path to recovery, take some time and consider each step. Make a concerted effort to do Step One and to feel the power behind it. Each step brings welcome and unexpected changes.

The best way to understand the Twelve Steps is to get help with them. Go to a beginner's AA or NA meeting where they cover Steps One through Three. Find a temporary sponsor and ask for help. Once we begin to better grasp the Steps and see the change in our lives, we want more. We need to allow ourselves time to get to that point. Everyone is different. We can't predict how long it will take to get through the Steps, but the more help you have, the better.

Following are some different avenues you can take to get help with your step work: a sponsor, step meetings, Twelve Step literature, and online help (use your search engine to find more detailed information about each step).

THE FENCE POSTS

We've learned that there is hope for a new life and that by truly embracing these Twelve Steps and performing the actions prescribed in each, we acquire a set of principles, not on our own but with the guidance of a sponsor. Think of these principles as fence posts, boundaries, encircling you in early recovery. Each fence post has a name: Honesty. Trust. Faith. Integrity. Courage. Justice. Perseverance. These fence posts create a corral where you can feel protected in early recovery; and within these boundaries, there is room enough for you, your sponsor, and your Higher Power. And in time, if the principles are practiced on a daily basis, the area expands, allowing room for other recovering people and perhaps, in time, your own sponsees.

If you step outside these boundaries and into the area where your character defects exist—beyond the fence post marked *honesty* into the area of dishonesty or beyond the fence post marked *courage* into an area of fear—that simply means you're human. Your awareness of that transgression allows you to get inside the safety of your recovery area as soon as you recognize that you have stepped outside of it. If you choose, for whatever reason, to remain outside of those protected boundaries, you can find yourself in the area of relapse, where your thinking begins to deteriorate and your attitude moves away from recovery and toward the action of drinking or using.

The Twelve Steps have given me both the foundation and boundaries that were missing in my life. Boundaries are the guideposts for a new and exciting life filled with predictable and cherished pleasure that I can share with those I love in a way I never thought possible. In being able to understand and embrace the Twelve Steps, we are truly blessed. We live in a life of anticipation of the next miracle rather than in fear of the next catastrophe.

— TAKEAWAYS —

» Drug and alcohol use damages the brain.

» In early recovery, we have trouble thinking clearly.

» Unable to think clearly, we may not grasp the Twelve Step message right away.

» Understanding the Twelve Steps is imperative to recovery.

» For now we can refer to the simplified version of the Steps provided in this chapter.

» We can get help with the Steps by attending meetings and finding a sponsor.

CHAPTER 6

SPIRITUAL AWAKENING (STOP YAWNING!)

"To undertake a genuine spiritual path is not to avoid difficulties but to learn the art of making mistakes wakefully, to bring them to the transformative power of our heart."

—JACK KORNFIELD

IT WAS HALLOWEEN during the '70s, and I was looking forward to a party at the home of a friend. Like most well-planned events back then, this one had a large stock of alcohol, along with the standard variety of contraband that included pills, powders, and smokes. I was dressed as a sheikh, and our host came to the door dressed in a turtleneck and jacket, sporting a full beard and a werewolf wig. He set a hilarious mood that only improved as other guests began arriving in outrageous costumes. Soul music, dancing, and colored lights in all the sockets created a festive and spooky atmosphere.

A buddy of ours got a little drunk before arriving that night. He decided at the last minute that the only thing he had to wear to the party was his brother's police uniform—not a costume but a legitimate uniform of the local police department. He arrived late; it was around 10:30 p.m., and the party was in full swing. He leaned on the doorbell while banging on the door with a billy club. "Open up," he said. "Police." Thinking this was going to be a hilarious spoof on all of us, he proceeded to open the door.

As the "cop" entered through the front door, about 50 percent of the party made their way into every available bathroom. I can't tell you how much of that contraband ended up flushed down toilets as panic, instead of drugs, raced through the veins of the would-be stoned. Drunken, raucous laughter followed as our costumed friend shouted, "Trick or treat!" Then someone fell into the turntable, creating a deafening screech as the needle dug into and across whatever record album was playing. Next came a hush of silence. The party was over. I can't even imagine who might have gotten hurt that evening or who might have done something terrible to someone else if all that stuff that was so suddenly flushed away had been consumed. God does indeed work in mysterious ways.

The Twelve Step program is spiritual in nature and has worked for millions of recovering people. Why, you might ask, does a spiritual program help us with a medical condition—a brain disease? Addiction is a complex disorder. We learned in Chapter 1 that it affects us physically, mentally, emotionally, and spiritually. Most of us have used alcohol or drugs to fill a void—an emptiness inside—whether or not we are religious. The spiritual nature of the Twelve Step program helps us fill that void naturally, without drugs or alcohol. By working the Steps, we experience a spiritual awakening. This does not necessarily mean we become Holy Rollers or start our own ministry (or even that we need to attend church regularly). A spiritual awakening is a shift in perception. Sometimes this shift is large and profound. Most times, it's subtle and may even happen piecemeal. How we experience a spiritual awakening is less important than the changes that result. Once we've stopped our spiritual yawning, we wake up. We can begin to live again.

SEEING THE LIGHT

Bill W., cofounder of AA, experienced a profound spiritual awakening. On his knees in a hospital room, praying to be relieved of his addiction, he saw and felt the warmth of a bright white light. Immediately afterward, his desire to drink had been lifted.

Everyone experiences a spiritual awakening in his or her own unique way. Most people do not see a bright white light. Many of us may feel a subtle shift in consciousness or a sudden (and foreign) feeling of joy in our gut.

SPIRITUALITY DEFINED

Spirituality can be loosely defined as a connection, and, like gravity, it is all around us all the time. Always present and exerting an effect.

What varies is our awareness of it, our acceptance of it, and our use of it. Spirituality is the quality of our relationship with whomever or whatever is most important to us. This includes the quality of the relationship we have with our Higher Power, our spouse, our co-workers, and our friends. And spirituality is also the quality of the relationship we have with ourselves—our goals and priorities, our values, and our preoccupations. If we are nurturing, caring, loving, trusting, and committed in our relationships, we bring a spiritual quality to them. If we are the opposite, we instantly lose the higher connection as shame, remorse, and fear block us from our spirituality and from experiencing the presence of our Higher Power. Therefore, spirituality is a part of our everyday life—it is a part of our makeup.

On any given day, our spiritual focus might make our relationships more or less caring. Even drugs and alcohol can be a spiritual focus, and when chemicals are the center of our spiritual focus, addiction becomes a spiritual disease.

A DIFFERENT KIND OF LOVE AFFAIR

For addicts, the relationship with alcohol or drugs becomes too important, a distraction. It commands all our attention to the detriment of other relationships. It draws energy, becomes a burden, and, as our focus on it grows, excludes family, friends, work, health, a Higher Power, and eventually life itself. I've heard it said by some that AA is a cultlike experience, but when we look at the devotion addicts who are active in their addiction give to their disease, we see how this disease commands all of the spiritual focus and attention of a love affair. Recovery demands the same level of devotion.

HIGHER POWER

When Bill W. and Dr. Bob founded AA back in the 1930s, before they wrote the Twelve Steps down on paper, they had already helped hundreds of alcoholics get into recovery. They were fully aware that some alcoholics were atheists or agnostics or grew up with a harsh image of a punitive God. They knew that not every religion believed in the same God, and they didn't care whether an addict believed in God at all. But they knew that their program worked because it was based on spiritual principles. They needed people to believe in a power greater than themselves, a spiritual power of some sort.

When it came time to write down the Twelve Steps, they used the language "God *as we understood Him*" to make it clear that they were talking about a spiritual power but how we envisioned that power was up to us. Like a beam of light, our spirituality needs to be focused on a relationship with an entity other than ourselves. We need to personalize it and make it a power we recognize, respect, and honor. A doorknob, a car, or other material item won't do—it's temporary and you have power over it.

Many people joke that their Higher Power is their spouse. But what we're looking for in a Higher Power is an energy that is much bigger and purer and more powerful than ours—God, the universal force, the energy that emanates from our home group.

Almost all of my patients speak of an inability to feel comfortable in their own skin or of a need to fill the hole in their gut. Something is missing. When alcohol or drugs fill that hole, we have, by definition, a spiritual disease, a spiritual problem. The comfort, decreased anxiety, and stress reduction that occur when we consume alcohol or other drugs, although very temporary, connect us to our drug of choice. Destructive spiritual relationships with alcohol or drugs develop when our experience with alcohol and drugs has satisfied some need: to be accepted, to combat boredom or loneliness, to fortify us with false perceptions of pride, to calm us, to motivate us, to change the way we feel, to give us a place to hide.

Every alcoholic and addict has experienced this. The shy may become outgoing; the weak may gain strength; the angry may become calmer; and the depressed, happier or forgetful. Throw genetics into the mix and, as we progress, we need our drugs or alcohol just to feel normal. We begin our journey into addiction in an honest attempt to feel happier, healthier, and safer. This is a common denominator in the stories of many who have the disease of addiction. Since our disease is of a spiritual nature, our drug of choice takes on God-like qualities in our quest for wholeness, overshadowing our other relationships with its progression.

A NEW DIRECTION FOR OUR SPIRITUAL FOCUS

In recovery, we redirect our spiritual focus. When we abstain from our chemicals and begin working the Twelve Steps, the image of ourselves clears and so does our image of the world around us. Some of this comes to us passively, but it also happens by our actions. We must be accountable and active participants in shifting our spiritual focus from drugs and alcohol to recovery. We begin by being truly *a part of* rather than *apart from* the process. Like a beam of light, our focus needs to be redirected to a new goal: abstinence and recovery one day at a time. The key to this shift is an open mind, a willing mind, and absolute rigorous honesty. We confront reality. We look at ourselves and allow accountability and participation in a Twelve Step Fellowship to get honest feedback. Sharing halves our burdens and doubles our joy.

FOUR BASIC SHIFTS

A change of spiritual focus results in a change of lifestyle. Our sanity is restored. Remember that spirituality deals with relationships, which can be positive or negative. Even a gang member can have a spiritual relationship with other gang members and have his needs met, though often in a negative way, by his gang and its activities. In order to move toward spirituality and maintain it in a positive light during recovery, we need to concentrate on four basic shifts: (1) fear to trust, (2) self-pity to gratitude, (3) resentment to acceptance, and (4) dishonesty to absolute rigorous honesty.

Fear to Trust

A life governed by fear is self-destructive: fear of finding out who we are, fear of intimacy, fear of offending others, fear of stating our needs. We can recognize fear by knowing some of the common physical symptoms: holding our breath, a queasy feeling in our stomach, a rapid pounding heartbeat, a clenched fist. These physical symptoms, even feelings of pain, are often messages that signal our fears. Often fears go unrecognized; we have to learn to scan ourselves, to find our fears and the ways they sometimes hide in other symptoms. Anger is often an emotional expression of fear— fear coming out sideways. We might be afraid we are going to lose our job and with it our financial security. The fear is so strong it has to find a way out somehow. When another driver cuts us off on our way home from work, we explode with rage.

To move from fear to trust, we identify our fears, expose them, and let people know who we are. We make ourselves vulnerable. We learn to know the difference between fears that make our body go into temporary stress mode to help ensure our survival (I see a grizzly bear ahead, and I need to decide whether to flee, fight, or freeze) and fears that turn us into nervous wrecks on an ongoing basis (I'm afraid I'm going to lose my job, and I can't stop worrying about it).

Self-Pity to Gratitude

As long as gratitude is a chore, we will make little progress. It's easy to be grateful for the bonus we got or the good meal on our plate. It is difficult for us to want to be grateful for our problems and our adversities. But every negative has a positive, and our job is to look for it. These problems allow us to cope, to become better people, and, in turn, to change our lives. Being grateful is really quite easy to do. One of the easiest methods of finding gratitude is to pray for people we resent. We can also thank our Higher Power for the people and situations that make us feel sorry for ourselves. In the shift from self-pity to gratitude, we reap benefits from even the slightest move in this positive direction. We can also try to remember the last negative consequence from our drinking or using and then recall what a single day without a negative consequence is like. Gratitude sets us free.

Resentment to Acceptance

We learn through trust and gratitude that acceptance is to take or receive willingly—that is, without judgment. When we accept people and situations as they are, we stop resisting what is and we stop trying to make it what we want it to be. We give up trying to control what isn't ours to control. With acceptance, we no longer need to feel pain or regret over and over. Acceptance is not about being right or wrong. It's not about being weak or giving in. Acceptance is about giving up the need to control people or situations and understanding that, in reality, we never really had control to begin with. Moving from resentment to acceptance (which usually starts with our Fourth Step inventory) produces a profound sense of relief. Trying to control that which is not controllable takes a great amount of energy, and releasing that burden is enormously satisfying.

Dishonesty to Absolute Rigorous Honesty

We cannot put our world together through external manipulation and control. We need to do some internal work. Integrity flows from trust, gratitude, and acceptance. Integrity makes wholeness and congruity of our beliefs and our actions. It is not possible to enjoy the glow of integrity without absolute honesty in all of our affairs. When I started to have that spiritual awakening and pray on a regular basis, I began seeing dishonesty turn to honesty, despair turn to hope, and self-pity turn to gratitude. It was only then that I finally began to focus back on recovery. That's the missing spiritual component I was able to find.

MAKING THE SHIFTS

The Twelve Steps give us the tools we need to create the four basic shifts, but the strength of our spirituality is only as good as the relationship we have with ourselves, others, and our Higher Power. The best way to start the shift is to establish or strengthen our relationship with our Higher Power. We do this by praying or meditating: We ask our Higher Power for help, and we admit that we cannot do this alone. We acknowledge that the power of alcohol and drugs has hijacked our brain. If we ask for humility and grace, the healing will flow. We must always invite that healing and never refuse it. We ask for our Higher Power to remove all obstacles.

Attending Twelve Step meetings, where we connect with others in the program, is our next best tool. In Chapter 7, we'll talk about the importance of attending meetings and share some ideas for how to get started.

— TAKEAWAYS —

» Spiritual awakenings are not always dramatic events, but they are powerful nonetheless.

» A spiritual awakening can be a subtle change in perception or a feeling of joy.

» Working the Steps brings us to a spiritual awakening.

» Spirituality is the quality of our relationship with whoever or whatever is most important to us. Spirituality is part of everyday life.

» Drugs and alcohol fill a spiritual void.

» In recovery, we redirect our spiritual focus.

» A change in spiritual focus results in a change in lifestyle.

» We make four basic shifts: fear to trust, self-pity to gratitude, resentment to acceptance, and dishonesty to honesty.

CHAPTER 7

THE CULTURE OF RECOVERY: WORKING THE PROGRAM

"You know you're an alcoholic when you misplace things—like a decade."

—Paul Williams

IT WAS A mild and very dark night when my nearly empty plane landed at the Hilton Head airport. I entered the tiny terminal, retrieved my luggage, and walked outside. I had been anticipating this golf trip for weeks and was excited to meet up with my buddies, who had planned all kinds of outlandish adventures. I knew I had a problem with alcohol (I hadn't had a drink in 5 years), but I was totally convinced that I could *probably* control it in my life. I was planning to reintroduce myself into the nightlife scene with my friends.

Parked curbside was a battered, old Chevrolet station wagon with a fly-spattered taxi sign on top. A large man sat behind the steering wheel, glasses down on his nose, reading a newspaper in the dimly lit interior. I got in the backseat, told him the name of my hotel, and asked whether he could wait for me while I checked in and then take me out to meet my buddies. I was ready to storm the beaches of Normandy, adrenaline coursing through my veins. He said, "No problem."

We drove off slowly in his creaky, old wagon. He introduced himself as Tom and spoke to me in a beautiful Southern drawl, encouraging me to talk about my life and history during the short drive. He learned I was a physician from Vermont who hadn't had a drink in a long time. Tonight, I told him, I had some great plans to meet up with my buddies, and I named the places we were supposed to go. He knew them all well. Oh, boy, did he know them well. He described a couple to me, saying I was probably in for a good old time. "Don't know about tomorrow, though," he said. "Might not be so much fun."

I barely heard that comment as we pulled up to the hotel. I ran in, changed my clothes, and jumped back into the cab. Tom said, "Okay, son, you ready to let it rip?"

"Let's let 'er rip!"

He pulled up to a darkened strip mall. Around the side stood a set of stairs, like a fire escape—you know, the metal kind you can see through. They went up in one direction and curved at a landing to a solitary door. One light hung over the top of the stairs. He said, "Well, Doc, here you go."

"Well, I'll be," I said. My buddies had gotten a private club—over a strip mall. I had no idea what we were going to do in there, but I assumed they had it all planned.

Tom said, "There'll be a couple of ladies up there to greet you." My pulse sped up a bit as I scurried up the stairs.

William L. White, historian and addictions specialist, defines culture as "a way of life, a means of organizing one's daily existence, and a way of viewing people and events in the outside world." In a culture of addiction, a group of people might share the viewpoint that getting drunk or high is fun and exciting and that being sober is a drag or that going to AA or treatment is like going to a cult. If we change the lens (the mind-set of the group) to that of promoting sobriety, we find ourselves in a culture of recovery. In this culture, the viewpoint is that sobriety and recovery bring us a full and meaningful life and that getting drunk or high is ruinous and deadly, at least for the addict.

RECOVERY IS COOL

Maybe you don't think the Twelve Steps sound very appealing. Maybe you don't think recovery sounds that great. Well, let's think about what happens with addiction: losing control; slurring your speech; being violent or aggressive; getting arrested; ruining your health; breaking the hearts of family and loved ones; spending too much money; putting yourself and others in harm's way; and wantonly and recklessly pushing aside principles, morals, and people to satisfy a hijacked brain. That doesn't sound so cool to me.

Now, think about a quiet, humble dignity; a soft, spiritual connection; and a palpable, caring, and nurturing relationship with others in your life. To be respected, to be honored, and to be loved and feel worthy of it. To know that you are worthwhile and to feel the joy of helping others. Recovery is cool. *Very* cool.

Cultures are strong influences, which is why staying clean and sober requires that we transition to a culture of recovery. When we make a conscious effort to abstain from drugs or alcohol, we meet and hang out with like-minded people—people who have the disease of addiction and who understand how to help us stay in recovery. We leave behind the other culture—the people, places, and things that can convince us that drinking or using offers us a better life. When our recovery is solid, some of us can safely return to the people and places of our former life and still maintain a clean and sober viewpoint. Some of us never have a reason to go back.

DROP THE ATTITUDE

When we hear others speak at Twelve Step meetings, the goal is to identify with the person and his or her story. The important word is *identify*, which is quite different from *compare*. Many people who have sat in a speaker meeting and listened to a drunkalogue have said to themselves, "Good Lord, I was never that bad," or, "Oh, WTF, listen to her! How could she have done such things?" These kinds of comparisons keep us from immersing ourselves into the group and discovering the magic that Bill W. and Dr. Bob found in 1935 when they founded the program—the magic of one alcoholic *identifying* with another, of knowing that if we haven't gone that far yet, this is what our disease has in store for us. And, if we have gone that far, it reminds us that we don't want to go back there again. We hear stories about the enormous toll the disease has taken on others—the jail time, the ER trips, the relapses—so that we do not have to do the research ourselves. We listen and hopefully we learn.

This shift to a culture of recovery takes some getting used to. If we decide to commit to the Steps, we need to work the program. That's right—*work*. Our weekly workload involves a mixture of fun, discipline, and action. It looks a little like this:

- Attend Twelve Step meetings.

- Maintain regular contact with a sponsor (and, eventually, with a sponsee).

- Work on one of the Steps.

- Take a daily moral inventory and make any necessary amends.

- Pray and meditate.

At first this sounds like a big time commitment. But if we think back, we realize we spent just as much time on destructive activities when actively using. Twelve Step work replaces that destructive "work" with positive work. Instead of going to a bar, we go to Twelve Step meetings. Instead of meeting our dealer, we visit with our sponsor. Instead of calculating how to get more of our drug, we figure out how to become a better person. We immerse ourselves in a culture of recovery.

TWELVE STEP MEETINGS: THE BUILDING BLOCK

The Twelve Step meeting is the basic building block of the program. Attending Twelve Step meetings is how we get involved and participate. Meetings are where we begin to weave the principles of the Twelve Steps into our lives and where we grow to understand the culture of recovery. Here we find the safety to share and identify (as opposed to "compare") with other alcoholics and addicts. Here we are exposed to new friends and a new social life.

The Twelve Step meeting is our introduction into a new culture of recovery, a culture where we will be not only rehabilitated but rehumanized. Here we learn to conduct our lives with the direction of a Higher Power and to care for and nurture ourselves and others for the common good of the Twelve Step Fellowship. We find a new social life that involves meetings before and after the Twelve Step meeting: small suppers, coffee and dessert, one-on-ones in the hallways where one alcoholic or addict bonds with another in an intimate fashion, sharing concerns and seeking help. We learn the tools of the program, reaching out to give and to ask for help and making ourselves available for service. Simple acts like sweeping a room, setting up chairs, and making coffee take on new importance. They become a symbol of our willingness to embrace the humility that is so vitally necessary to receive the gift of recovery and to hold on to it so we can share it and pass it on to others.

The Twelve Step meeting is almost always where we find a sponsor—someone who understands the disease of addiction and whom we can trust to help us; someone who is available, accountable, open-minded, willing to help, and vulnerable. A sponsor is someone who makes us feel nurtured, cared for, and truly worthwhile. A sponsor is there for us when we need direction, a helping hand, or a lifeline. A sponsor is someone we can share our worries and our big and small successes with. Having a sponsor is vital to our recovery, and one of the best ways to find a sponsor is at a Twelve Step meeting.

WHAT IS A SPONSOR, AND WHY DO I NEED ONE?

A sponsor is someone with at least 2 years of solid recovery under his or her belt who helps us work through the program. Our sponsor is our touchstone—someone we call when we have a craving so we can talk it through. Someone we meet with for coffee and a movie on a Saturday evening, when our other friends are out partying. Our sponsor should be our same gender. We should feel comfortable talking to our sponsor about anything. We can look for a sponsor at a Twelve Step meeting. We single out someone we think we can relate to and, after a meeting, simply ask if he or she will sponsor us. A good sponsor picks up the phone when we call or returns our calls promptly, listens to our story, and is able to apply Twelve Step philosophy to our situation. Our sponsor is our central support person—the one we go to when those close to us who aren't in recovery won't understand. Without a sponsor, we are left to our own devices.

TYPES OF MEETINGS

The Twelve Steps are the foundation for many different groups, including Alcoholics Anonymous, Narcotics Anonymous, Al-Anon (for family members), Alateen, Gamblers Anonymous, Sex Addicts Anonymous, and so on. Each group offers different types of meetings. It may take some trial and error before we find the meetings that are right for us. Most meetings are about 1 to 2 hours long. Some meetings are open (anyone can attend regardless of whether they're in the program). Other meetings are closed, or for members only. The most important meeting is probably our home group.

Home Group

A home group is just what it sounds like—the meeting where we feel most at home. By default, it is the meeting we frequent most. Our home group can be any kind of meeting—Step, specialty, Big Book. We sit in the same chair, if possible—not in the "denial aisle," or the back row, but up front where we can pay attention, become engaged, and connect by looking into the eyes of a speaker. We add our phone number to the home group sheet. We get to know other attendees. We feel at home. Truly an essential part of the program, our home group is where a community of relationships blossoms. There's something about sitting in a diner over lunch with a home group member and knowing that tonight

CHANGING SPONSORS

What do we do if we think we picked the wrong sponsor? We don't want to hurt anyone's feelings by "rejecting" them, but at the same time, we need a sponsor who we feel can help us. Our first step is to review what is working. Perhaps our sponsor is always available when we need him and always calls if he has to cancel an engagement. Then we need to understand what isn't working. Is it an age difference? A communication issue? Have we outgrown the help our sponsor can offer us? Then we must ask ourselves what we *do* want in a sponsor. If we're going to get rid of the old one, we need to know what qualities we need in our new one. Lastly, we need to inform our sponsor of our decision. The answers to the questions above give us the content we need for our conversation: We tell him what he does well and what we're wanting from a sponsor. We keep it honest and positive. Most sponsors will understand.

or tomorrow night we'll be sitting at a Twelve Step meeting together—the discussion immediately goes to a deeper level. The intimacy that's fostered in the Twelve Step program is a spiritual connection among its members who are practicing the principles of honesty, open-mindedness, and willingness.

Specialty Groups

When it's time to suit our Twelve Step program more closely to our personal needs, we find a specialty, or "special," group. For example, we may go to a men's group or a women's group, a group based on sexual persuasion, a young person's group, or a group for the elderly. There are professional groups for health care professionals, lawyers, and pilots. A doctor, for example, can get honest in an entirely different way in a room with a group of doctors. If he's stealing pills from his nursing home patients, the safest place to reveal that secret is among his professional peers who have a better chance of understanding all the circumstances. It's much safer than trying to do that in a meeting where he may be sitting next to a bodybuilder whose mother lives in a nursing home. These groups are not the main focus of the program. It is not about boxing ourselves into a niche where we feel too special or different; it is about intensifying the program with those who may understand certain special aspects of our life and those with whom we might identify a bit more closely. Sponsors can be vital in guiding us in finding these types of groups.

Step Meetings

One of the most important and most overlooked meetings is a weekly Step meeting. Step meetings give us the opportunity to learn as much as we can about each step. They're also a place to "take a Step," or to present our Step work in a formal fashion to the group and to get feedback. Because some of the subjects are highly personal, they are best done in a gender-specific group. The same group of men or women meets weekly. I've known men who have taken their Twelve Steps formally six, seven, or more times in their recovery and each time gotten new feedback and a new perspective from the group. They see the progress that the program promises when they put in the work.

90/90

Conventional recovery wisdom dictates that, upon discharge, newcomers to the program should attend 90 meetings in 90 days. Sponsors often issue this same exercise to sponsees who've relapsed. There may be something to this 90-day exercise and its ability to cultivate some good habits. But, truth be told, I have observed some people greatly reduce the number of meetings they attend after their 90-day trial. They've met their goal, and now they're done. I prefer that newcomers embrace three or four meetings per week that they simply wouldn't want to live without—meetings that are personalized and special for them. This typically includes a variety of meetings such as a speaker meeting or a discussion meeting, a Step meeting, a Big Book meeting, and perhaps a specialty group meeting. Remember: This is your program, and you can customize it to work for you. Embrace it as a personal gift.

Speaker, Open, or Discussion Meetings

The speaker meeting, also known as an open meeting or discussion meeting, is what most people think of when they hear "Twelve Step meeting." During the first half of a speaker meeting, members share how they came to AA or NA, what it has done for them, and why they keep coming back. The speakers are usually guests from other home groups. The last half of the meeting involves discussion. These meetings serve the important purpose of reminding us where we came from and give us deeper insight into the role of the Twelve Steps in our recovery. They are only helpful, however, if we identify with the speakers. If we don't identify, we leave feeling that we're different. The easiest way to identify with the speakers is to avoid comparing our experiences to theirs.

Big Book Meetings

Big Book meetings can be open or closed. At these meetings, each person reads a paragraph or two from the Big Book aloud. (We can just say "pass" if we don't want to read aloud.) Typically, at the end of each chapter, the group discusses what they just read and how they can relate to the information. The Big Book meeting can be likened to a Bible study group in that it helps us learn how to interpret the stories and other information in the text.

What to Avoid

It is quite possible to select meetings where we will not have to participate. That's a dangerous practice. Attending only speaker meetings (however fascinating or meaningful they may be) does not allow the vital participation in the Fellowship that keeps us sober. Because the opposite sex can be distracting, one of your group meetings should be gender specific.

GETTING TO YOUR FIRST MEETING

Before you can go to a meeting, you need to find one. If you're already in treatment, your counselor can recommend local meetings (and maybe already has). If you're not yet in treatment, call the Alcoholics Anonymous headquarters in New York at 212-870-3400, or go online and visit www.aa.org for a meeting locator. Narcotics Anonymous, based in Los Angeles, can be reached at 818-773-9999 or at www.na.org. You might also consider purchasing a Twelve Step app that can help you find meetings when you're on the road or traveling out of state. These sources can also provide you with information about online meetings, which are becoming more and more popular and offer additional confidentiality.

Now, write down the meeting(s) you plan to start with and the date and time you plan to go: _____

_____

_____

_____.

Write down the address and directions:

_____

_____

_____

_____.

Now forget about it. That's right. Forget about the meeting and instead focus on making a contract with yourself. Even if you're not there already, aim to be someone who follows through. Write down your promise to yourself—your promise to go to this first meeting and to go at least five times. (If you find you don't like the meeting you've chosen for whatever reason, you can change locations. Just stick with your promise to yourself to attend at least five meetings in one location.)

I promise . . .

_____

_____

_____

_____

Remember, there are no membership dues, and you don't need to make an appointment or reserve a seat. You just need to show up. And the best part is that, when you do show up, people will be glad you came.

PREPARING FOR YOUR FIRST TWELVE STEP MEETING

Walking into a meeting for the first time can be daunting. Newcomers don't always know what to expect. Most don't want to be there. Most don't think they need to be there. And most go in not planning to return. Given that you're aiming for 90 meetings in 90 days (or at least three or four quality meetings every week), it's important that you know what to expect from yourself and from others. The first meeting can help to prepare you for the experience.

Why do we go to Twelve Step meetings?

We go to meetings to find a safe environment where we can begin to practice the principles of the Steps. Saying out loud "I'm Joe and I'm an alcoholic" may be the first time we've practiced the First Step principle of honesty in a long time. Meetings are also a social experience for us. We need to make sure we laugh and don't take things too seriously. People at Twelve Step meetings are fun to be with, and we will get some of the benefits from an AA meeting that we got from going to a bar, except we don't get handcuffed at the end of the night. In addition, by participating in meetings and being in a healthy social environment, we are lighting up some of the areas of the brain that counter some of the cognitive damage from drinking or using.

Why is it that a Twelve Step meeting will sometimes turn people off?

We feel uncomfortable and as if we don't belong at a meeting when we start to compare ourselves to the other people at the meeting. We need to be able to identify with them, and the best way to do that is to keep an open mind. If we go into a meeting dead set against it and everyone associated with it, we're bound to be turned off by it. A good plan is to promise ourselves that we're going to arrive on time, stay until the end, and try each meeting at least five times. At that point, we can see if we need to look somewhere else. One time at one meeting is not enough.

For our first meeting, it's best to go with someone we trust. Feeling a lot of anxiety and being with people we can't identify with is not the best way to start out. We need to be sure to identify ourselves as newcomers to give people the opportunity to welcome us. If we say nothing else, we can at least raise ourselves and tell the group our

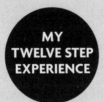

MY TWELVE STEP EXPERIENCE

To better understand how you feel about Twelve Step meetings, answer the following questions:

1. Have you ever been to any type of Twelve Step meeting before (AA, NA, Al-Anon, Gamblers Anonymous)?
2. If no, why not?
3. If yes, how many times did you go?
4. How did you feel before going to each meeting?
5. How did you feel during the meeting?
6. How did you feel the next morning?
7. Did you want to go back?
8. Do you feel you gave it your best effort?
9. What's your attitude about Twelve Step meetings now?
10. How can you improve your attitude?

name, that we've had some problems with alcohol or drugs, that we're here to listen and could use some help. The important thing is not to bail out before the miracle happens.

What do I look for in a meeting?

Look for the magic, the feeling of belonging, that longing to return. Evidence shows that some form of therapy combined with Twelve Step meetings is the solution to our disease. It took some time, but in 1998, Project MATCH, one of the largest studies to support Twelve Step philosophy, concluded that support meetings do have a positive effect on long-term sobriety. It may take a few tries to find the right one, but it's well worth the effort. If we don't make these efforts, we are inviting our disease to take over again.

Alcoholics Anonymous and Narcotics Anonymous are just that—meetings where we can remain anonymous. When we enter a meeting room, we'll probably find some people making coffee, some people in conversation, and others sitting alone and not talking to anyone. Some people will acknowledge us with a nod, a smile, or a hello. Others will walk right past us. When the time comes to share, we don't have to say anything. We don't have to stand up, share our name, and admit that we're a drug addict. We

---

ACT LIKE A NEWBIE

During early recovery, it's wise to act like a newcomer. When we think of ourselves as newbies, there's no expectation to know everything. We know nothing and need to learn everything. Being humble in this regard is the safest, highest ground. It beats relapsing because we think we know it all.

don't have to hug anyone. We don't have to recite any prayers. We don't have to sign any contracts or pay any membership fees. We don't even have to listen.

When we leave the meeting, even if we didn't actively partici-pate, we might be surprised by how uplifted we feel and decide that we're looking forward to going to the next meeting. Or we might be angry. We might be stewing about missing Monday night football. We might think that none of what these crazy people are saying applies to us. This is the disease's powerful defense mechanism. It gives us an unlimited number of reasons why the program isn't for us. This is why we want those four or five unbeatable meetings per week. In time, addiction's defense mechanisms weaken.

After the first 90 days, whether we've done a meeting a day or four or five per week, some of us think we've met our goal and can relax. Beware this kind of thinking. It's important not to jump off the bus in 90 days. We must be diligent. Ideally, we stick with our four or five unbeatable meetings per week. Our meetings are our medicine. If we neglect to take our medicine, our disease resurfaces.

I personally had a lot of trouble understanding the importance of meetings. My counselor had me write down my entire miserable life, admit that it was governed by selfish motives, self-pity, and resentment, and then tell that to someone I trusted. I had to con-front the facts and decide whether I wanted to live like that any longer. It wasn't until I finally got to the first of the Twelve Steps—the one that I like to paraphrase as "There is a power that wants to kill me"—that I was forced to be honest and to draw from the trough of shame. I didn't realize that my shame had been disguising itself as anger, arrogance, and self-importance. All shame-based, and I was never a big believer in shame. I liked guilt better. I understood it and knew I could do something about it. I had the Eighth and Ninth Steps to help me make amends with those things I felt guilty about.

The truth is that in the recovery I have today and because of the support I find in my meetings, I can now access that shame from my past, work with it, and finally come out from under the dark cloak and into light to do one of the most sacred things that a human being can possibly do: *ask for help*. How am I able to ask for help when my whole life has been about people asking me for help? I have to say, "I have to stop doing this. I'm going to have to put up some boundaries and trust someone else, trust my Higher Power." It really is a sacred process to ask for help and to be asked for help. It's what Alcoholics Anonymous and people have taught me—that I certainly can't do this alone.

MAKING THE MOST OF EACH MEETING

By attending meetings regularly, we become part of a Fellowship—we join the company of equals and friends. Participation in the Fellowship supports and nurtures some important qualities, including honesty (as we listen to others tell the truth about their addiction) and spirituality (as we feel connected to others in the Fellowship). Honesty is essential in admitting our mistakes and embracing our shortcomings. Through the connection we have in the Fellowship, we develop accountability to ourselves and to others. Here we develop a sense of ownership in our meetings and become *a part of* rather than *apart from*. Often this leads to service work both in the group and in the organization as a whole. Our daily work becomes the work of surrender, asking for help and guidance and reaching out to help others. We use prayer and meditation to cultivate spiritual awareness. We look at the character defects in our lives, expose them, share them, and turn them over to our Higher Power for their removal in our lives today.

After meetings, we may choose to journal or do a Tenth Step to seek balance and to clean up our own personal wreckage from the day. An obsessive lifestyle leads to loss of self. A balanced lifestyle embraces mental and spiritual health and a balance of intimacy and dependency with others. Removal of the obsession to drink or use from our lives, one day at a time, reaps the gifts of new relationships.

The Fellowship reminds us that addiction replaces human bonding and caring. We remember the adage "Only you alone can do it, but you cannot do it alone." In the program, we seek the happy balance of a purposeful life. Careful self-examination, sharing, and wide-open feedback alert us to feelings of entitlement, especially when we are physically and emotionally overextended. From this vantage point, we're able to observe cravings, obsessive thinking, the return of denial, euphoric recall (a process where we pretty up our past to make it more acceptable and palatable in the present), poor coping abilities, bad decision making and problem solving, and unsafe behavior.

Our work in the program prepares us for the inevitable stresses unique to our daily lives. Some of us went to bars and drank to find happiness, fellowship, camaraderie, and understanding. In our culture of addiction, we went to our drinking or partying buddies to help us solve problems and make decisions only to find that it created more problems or worsened our dilemmas. In our culture of recovery, the Twelve Step meeting is where we find clean and sober friends who help us without the adverse consequences, bathing us in a new light of grace that guides us from one day to the next. In the end, the

Twelve Step meeting should provide us with a sense of fellowship, acceptance, and love we never imagined possible with a night out with the boys or the girls. There are no hangovers from Twelve Step meetings, only the lingering feeling of joy.

KEEP COMING BACK

Using a one-day-at-a-time, keep-it-simple model works. This is an approach where we can see the little things early, the little things that can add up to big trouble in the life of the alcoholic or the addict. Through the program, we also develop the simple daily habits that support the discipline of good recovery.

Addicts and alcoholics need structure, and the program offers exactly that: We are doing it and living it, not just *knowing* or *studying* it. The program helps us define our personal behaviors that can indicate a return to imbalance. Attending meetings regularly is essential, for this cunning and baffling disease will reactivate if we provide it with space in our lives. But all the meetings in the world can't keep you sober unless you're working a program.

— TAKEAWAYS —

» Culture is a way of life, a way of viewing the world.

» In recovery, we shift from a culture of addiction to a culture of recovery.

» Twelve Step meetings are helpful building blocks of recovery.

» Twelve Step meetings provide us with a safe environment to begin to practice the principles of the Steps.

» We attend a meeting at least five times before we decide whether we like it or not.

» At a meeting, we avoid comparing ourselves to others and instead identify with others.

» The goal is to attend four or five different meetings every week.

» Our home group is the meeting we frequent most often.

» It's important to keep coming back.

I REACHED THE top of the stairs and found a curious name on the door. It read "Yana." Odd name for a club, I thought. Never heard of it before. I knocked on the door, it opened, and two ladies met me. One looked about 70 and the other one about 85, with curly, bluish-gray hair. They literally grabbed each of my hands and said, "We've been waiting for you, dahlin'. You're with Tom, arncha? Come right in!"

They led me over to a table where a cup of coffee waited for me alongside a plate of cookies, and before I knew it, a small white disk was placed in my hand. I still have that disk. It's called a newcomer's chip. Tom had dropped me off at the Yana Club, an Alcoholics Anonymous club in Hilton Head where you call ahead and have people wait around to hold a special meeting. He knew that if I relapsed that night, I could die. He knew that my plan was the work of the disease of alcoholism in my life. And he had the courage to call ahead and to make those arrangements while I was in the hotel.

Well, I sat down with those wonderful folks and they told me their stories. I soon loosened up and told them a little bit about myself. They all seemed in agreement that I was probably in the right place, and when our meeting was over, we all joined hands and said the Serenity Prayer.

On my way out, I asked them, "By the way, what does *Yana* stand for?" The older of the two ladies took my hand and looked me in the eye. Hers were sparkly blue and twinkling. "Yana stands for You Are Not Alone," she said.

I spent a glorious week with my friends; I played a lot of golf, had a wonderful time, and never picked up a drink. I never had the chance to thank him personally, so I'll do it here: Thank you, Tom.

CHAPTER 8

ONE DAY AT A TIME

"The best thing about the future is that it comes only one day at a time. Each day I got down on my knees because there was nowhere else to go."

—ABRAHAM LINCOLN

I ONCE SAT next to a nurse at an open Twelve Step meeting, which happened to be at a hospital. Attentive and observant, she remained silent during the meeting, clearly in a state of deep thought and concentration. When the meeting was over, I welcomed her and introduced myself. She made it clear she had never been to a Twelve Step meeting before and that she didn't have a problem with alcohol or drugs but just happened upon the meeting. She was impressed by what she'd heard and even more impressed by the Twelve Step concept. She was so in awe that she reiterated the concepts she'd learned during the meeting, just to be sure she had gotten it right.

"Now let me get this straight," she said. "You people believe you have a fatal disease. You believe you can push this disease into remission by not using and by practicing these steps posted on the wall. And if you don't drink or use drugs, no one will know you have this disease?"

"Yes," I said.

I'll never forget the nurse's response. It is perhaps the best antidote I have if I should ever take this program for granted. She said simply, "I have ovarian cancer and 3 to 6 months to live. Do you know what I would give to have the Twelve Steps for my disease?"

"One day at a time" is probably the most recognizable and most oft-quoted AA phrase ever—to the point of being cliché. But many recovering individuals hang their sobriety on this one powerful phrase. To the newcomer, it means simply, "I only have to stay sober for the next 24 hours. This I can do. This I can manage. It might not be easy, but I can get through one day without a drink or a hit." To the old-timer, one day at a time means, "Each day I clean my slate, through prayer and through Step work, so that when I wake in the morning, I start with a fresh clean slate—no resentments, no shame, no reason to drink or use. I do this every day, one day at a time."

Used on a daily basis, the Twelve Steps give us the fuel we need not just to get through the day without a drink but to enjoy it and then, as we get deeper and deeper into recovery, to live most of our days feeling content with ourselves and others. This is the power behind "one day at a time."

A CLEAN SLATE

When I ask a group of patients to list some of the feelings that flood through them before they are even out of bed in the morning, the list is enormous. It fills the clean slate—the large white eraser board at the front of the room. Fear. Dishonesty. Denial. Despair. Anxiety. Resentment. Unwillingness. Grandiosity. Suspicion. Procrastination. The list goes on and on—one word overlying another word. Soon the white of the eraser board is all but obliterated, choked by these assaults on the newfound sanity that we had hoped to carry with us throughout our day. These are the mushrooms that pop up in our lawns on a daily basis. Is it any wonder that our recovery is threatened on a daily basis? The stress that these unwelcome feelings places on us can only be met with firmly entrenched, malignant denial—a defense mechanism that, flimsy though it may be, allows us to accept ourselves and muddle through the day with this enormous burden. But we pay a price for these burdens.

The Twelve Step program shows us how to clean our slates, how to free ourselves from daily burdens that, in our using days, would have been reason enough to pick up a drink or a drug. A clean slate

A HEAVY LOAD

In the Betty Ford Center's Children's Program, each child is given a knapsack filled with heavy rocks. Painted on each rock is a word such as Anger, Fear, Doubt, Resentment, Loneliness, Exhaustion, Cockiness, or Irritability. After dragging the knapsack a few feet to feel its enormous weight, each child reaches into his or her knapsack and pulls out one stone. After it is read and discussed, it is left out of the bag. The kids learn about the enormous benefit that comes from recognizing and sharing these secret burdens, and they experience how it feels to lighten the load, to be cleansed, and to be granted that daily reprieve that we so desperately need to foster rich and fulfilling lives. They see and feel the burden carried by their addicted parents and themselves, and they learn firsthand how to deal with it instead of stuffing it back into the bag.

is a state of mind we have when we've taken proper care of our recovery business, a state of mind where we have no issues going on that could cause us anger or resentment. We use certain Twelve Step tools to take care of this business.

OUR DAILY REPRIEVE

When I was in early recovery, I heard someone say he had 15,000 days sober. I was fascinated by the way he kept track of his sobriety, and I never forgot that. If you hear someone say she's on her 8,654th day of sobriety, it tells you something about that person. It tells you that she approaches each day as a gift, and when she puts her head on her pillow at night, she places that gift back into the hands of her Higher Power. Each morning, the alcoholic prays again for that same gift. It's a 24-hour cycle of recovery, and it works.

The gift we have is recovery. Part of what recovery gives us is a reprieve. Webster's Dictionary defines reprieve as a "temporary respite from pain or trouble." We can look at it as temporary access to peace of mind. The key word here is *temporary*. Our daily reprieve is just that—a daily break from whatever ails us, from whatever thought or problem or anxiety might bring us down, give us false pride, compel us to control others or situations, or regurgitate old, harmful feelings and behaviors. We focus on obtaining this reprieve every day—sometimes morning, noon, night, and in between.

Imagine going to bed at night and saying a soft prayer or meditation, giving thanks for a day that was productive—filled with ups and downs that in the end seemed to work out. It was a day where family and friends survived, shared, loved, and cared; a day, perhaps, where some catastrophes beyond our control affected people we love, and we were able to help. And it was a day where our character defects rose and adversely affected a relationship. Now, if we worked our recovery during that day, we applied our Twelve Step tools. We prayed for awareness—for the ability to recognize the source of those relationship difficulties ideally at the time they occurred. We apologized to someone we might have offended or sought to clarify a point that, if left alone, could bring on smoldering resentment for us.

At the end of the day, we did the Tenth Step: We took the day's inventory; we listed our assets and our liabilities for the day. We were able to recognize when our "self-will run riot" crashed into the self-will of another individual. We realized that most of the difficulties encountered during the day were due to our lack of acceptance, and we rested easy, knowing we did something positive about it so the burden wasn't carried into a restful night's sleep or into the next day.

In the morning, we begin with the knowledge of who we are, with the serenity to accept the things we cannot change, with the courage to change the things we can, and with the wisdom to know

SELF-WILL RUN RIOT

"Self-will run riot" is a line from the Big Book. It describes the controlling and manipulative nature of many alcoholics and addicts. It's how we behave when we try to have things go our way. It's what we do when we don't accept people or events as they are and when we don't trust in our Higher Power. When this happens, we are driven by our character defects of fear, greed, and self-pity. In other words, we are hard to be around.

the difference. For all intents and purposes, we appear to start our day with a clean slate. Perhaps we do the Third Step prayer, asking that the will of our Higher Power be revealed to us and for relief from the bondage of self (you know, stop trying to be the big cheese). And maybe we do the Seventh Step prayer, asking for removal of our character defects today so we can embrace humility. And then we begin our day. We are out there in our lives. We plan our day: self-care, family, coworkers, schedules, deadlines, injunctions, and expectations. We take care of matters that, in the past, we would have handled poorly or ignored altogether (which would have given us an excuse to drink or use).   ·

One patient told me that the one-day-at-a-time approach gave him the option of drinking tomorrow. This option seemed to comfort him, to allow him relief from the enormous burden of the expectation that he had to make commitments today that were going to last the rest of his life. For him, that expectation did not seem to address his humanness—his vulnerabilities and his history—and he found that each day this was a contract that he could renew, a contract that brought enormous benefit not only to himself but to all those in his life.

One day at a time is a concept that works well for young people, who often have a sense of invincibility. How difficult it is to convince them that they need to embrace a habit today that needs to last for the rest of their lives. It's an unrealistic expectation, but to make it through 24 hours—outstanding! In recovery, we need to embrace a sense that we are the best custodians, along with our Higher Power, of our own lives. We need to take personal responsibility.

One way of thinking about our spirituality is to consider what it means to be a truly good human being. What separates us from animals? We can think about our personal history and take actions based on that history. We are capable of basing our thinking on morals and moral actions. We are able to forgive. And we have a conscious connection to a universal sense of being good for the betterment of the species. Applying the Twelve Step principles one day at a time naturally makes us stronger spiritually.

As we grow in recovery, the one-day-at-a-time approach morphs from "getting sober" to "staying sober" to "living life with a clean slate" to "unending days of joy and peace and discovering amazing, I-never-thought-possible experiences." Our desire to drink or use diminishes until it is a faint and distant memory—ancient history. The tools we use to seek our daily reprieve become a part of who we are, as natural and necessary as eating or bathing. Yet each new day is just as important as the last, approached with humility and care, approached as the gift it is.

Einstein's definition of insanity is doing the same thing over and over again and expecting different results. The best definition I've heard of faith is doing the same thing over and over again and expecting the same result. This gives us the confidence that we might make it to the end of the day. With faith, we start to live with less fear, and that faith comes from the Third Step.

A DAY IN THE LIFE OF A RECOVERING ADDICT

What are the tools we use every day, every 24 hours, to stay sober and sane? The program gives us many. Our greatest tool is communication with our Higher Power. We bookend our day with prayer and meditation and start a conversation with our Higher Power anytime we feel a need to during the day—when we feel like using, when we're unsure about how to handle an argument, when we feel hurt, when we hurt someone else's feelings, when we're dishonest, when we're grateful. From this, we receive awareness and we know the right action to take. Maybe we apologize, pray for another, or tell the truth. Our behavior, which is now aligned with our values, leaves us feeling neither righteous nor proud but full of peace and serenity.

The process goes something like this:

1. I wake up with a clean slate, having done a Tenth Step the night before.

2. I start the day with some prayer, meditation, and routine rituals of self-care—I make my bed, work out, take a shower, eat a healthy breakfast.

3. I begin the day's work—daily tasks and recovery. I may go to a meeting or have office work to do. If some unwelcome or untoward event rocks the boat, I do a midday Tenth Step. I might say the Third and Seventh Step prayers or the Serenity Prayer (see pages 142–43) and, in effect, start the day over. I apply the principles of awareness and acceptance, and I take the right action (which might be no action).

4. In the evening, I look at my day and review my Tenth Step list, my positive and negative actions, and add to it if necessary. This is an inventory, so I list both the good and the bad. I pray, I have a good night's sleep, and I start tomorrow with a clean slate.

Here is the 24-hour-day model I use for my patients: Four hours are specifically reserved for treatment of a disease whose presence is lifelong. One of those hours is used for a Twelve Step meeting. One hour is used for prayer, meditation, literature, journaling, and calls to sponsors and sponsees. One hour is used for maintenance of physical and mental health—working out, further meditation, a great walk—and 1 hour is for pure fun. We have to make this program fun. After all, this is what we sought in the substances that came back to bite us.

During the other 20 hours, we are required to get a good night's sleep—at least 7 or 8 hours—and adjust our day to accommodate family, employment, and service work. At first, this seems like a tall order, but it is possible. Like patience and tolerance, it takes practice.

We talk about shortcomings and character defects in the steps of this program. Those are powerful terms that address our self-pride. We need to be mindful that a defect does not necessarily always mean the presence of a bad thing. It may represent the lack of enough of a good thing. This was once demonstrated at an AA meeting by my friend Mike, who held up a napkin with a hole in the middle, showing a defect that simply meant a lack of enough of what was supposed to be there—more material to fill the hole.

We might have a lack of love, a lack of self-respect, a lack of confidence, or a lack of good humor. These might also be among the defects from which we need relief. A wonderful friend, Dr. Jim West, once told me, "Don't make the mistake of assuming that the character defects whose removal you pray for today will be removed tomorrow." They are removed for 1 day only. I have experienced the truth of his statement firsthand, watching them pop up again in my life like mushrooms on a lawn.

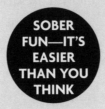

SOBER FUN—IT'S EASIER THAN YOU THINK

Fun is an essential part of a recovery program and needs to be instilled in your life each day. Having fun is easy. All you need is an open mind and a few ideas. If, after reading the following list, you're feeling cynical, try acting "as if." Act as if it's fun. Before long, it will be. And soon enough, you'll be creating your own list, one that suits your interests and lifestyle. Here are a few ideas to try:

1. *Learn new skills.* Create the best BBQ sauce recipe; bake an elaborate dessert; learn to knit or crochet; take a discover scuba class or dance lessons. Learning new skills, even simple ones, broadens your horizons and can make you feel great.

2. *Challenge your mind.* Work on crossword puzzles; play Words with Friends, Scrabble, or Sudoku; take a class; write a children's story and read it to a child. Challenging your mind improves your cognitive abilities—and it's fun.

3. *Get active.* Join a team sport or a health club, run, bike, ski, golf, bowl, walk. Try being a child for a day and make "play" your number one goal. The more physical you are, the more endorphins, or feel-good chemicals, your body releases and the better you feel.

4. *Get outdoors.* Garden, hike, walk, paint, fish, camp. Learn the names of wildflowers and trees. Go to a local Little League game. Fresh air and nature, plain and simple, will make you feel good and full of life.

5. *Volunteer.* Serve food at a soup kitchen; mow your neighbor's lawn; join a ski patrol; make coffee at your AA meeting; coach a team; seat patrons at a theater. Nothing helps you more than helping others.

6. *Relax.* Listen to music; watch a movie; stargaze; soak in a hot bath; read; write. Taking time for yourself is necessary and valuable. Enjoy it.

And of course go to meetings, meetings, meetings, and meet new people to share your experiences. Keep in mind that group activities are best done with sober people who are also in recovery. Without alcohol or drugs, we are still people, and we are much more fun when we're clean and sober.

PRAYERS

Following are some prayers commonly recited by those of us in recovery. Of course it's not necessary to pray or meditate using traditional, religious language, and you are free to amend any of these prayers or come up with your own mantras. But many patients find these prayers in particular very useful and comforting.

Third Step Prayer

God, I offer myself to Thee—to build with me and to do with me as Thou wilt. Relieve me of the bondage of self, that I may better do Thy will. Take away my difficulties, that victory over them may bear witness to those I would help of Thy Power, Thy Love, and Thy Way of life. May I do Thy will always!

Seventh Step Prayer

My Creator, I am now willing that you should have all of me, good and bad. I pray that you now remove from me every single defect of character which stands in the way of my usefulness to you and my fellows. Grant me strength, as I go out from here to do Your bidding.

THE GIFT

Recovery is a gift. Each day we get to open the safe, take it out of its special box to embrace it, polish it, appreciate it, and protect it. And at the end of each day, we place it back in the safe, back in the hands of our Higher Power for yet another day when we can pray for its return to our lives.

Serenity Prayer

God, grant me the serenity to accept the things I cannot change, courage to change the things I can, and the wisdom to know the difference. Living one day at a time; enjoying one moment at a time; accepting hardship as the pathway to peace. Taking, as He did, this sinful world as it is, not as I would have it. Trusting that He will make all things right if I surrender to His Will; that I may be reasonably happy in this life, and supremely happy with Him forever in the next.

Eleventh Step Prayer of St. Francis

Lord, make me a channel of thy peace, that where there is hatred, I may bring love; that where there is wrong, I may bring the spirit of forgiveness; that where there is discord, I may bring harmony; that where there is error, I may bring truth; that where there is doubt, I may bring faith; that where there is despair, I may bring hope; that where there are shadows, I may bring light; that where there is sadness, I may bring joy.

Lord, grant that I may seek rather to comfort than to be comforted; to understand, than to be understood; to love, than to be loved. For it is by self-forgetting that one finds. It is by forgiving that one is forgiven.

It is by dying that one awakens to Eternal Life.

Old wisdom has given us the one-day-at-a-time approach to recovery that seems to have sustained alcoholics and addicts for many, many years. The more I learned about this disease, the more things got better, one day at a time. Now, I tell my story to someone I really trust. Then, on a daily basis, I take a personal inventory, sometimes twice a day, so it doesn't get backed up. I make sure things are right. If they are not right, I go back and try to fix them.

When I started to get that spiritual awakening and to pray on a regular basis, I started to see dishonesty turn to honesty, despair turn to faith and trust, and my self-pity turn to gratitude. Only then was I able to turn my focus back to recovery. That's the spiritual change that I was able to find. It was in the refocusing.

HOW TO LIVE ONE DAY AT A TIME

Awareness, acceptance, and right action are all important concepts in living one day at a time using the Twelve Step program. The better understanding we have of these terms, the better we'll be able to live them and carry them out.

Awareness

Awareness is being conscious of what's happening around us, inside and out. When we're walking down the street and are aware of our surroundings, we're conscious of what businesses are open across the street, of who's walking behind us, and whether it's sunny or cloudy, warm or cold. We're aware of the expressions on people's faces.

On the inside, we are conscious of our feelings. Did something we just think, do, see, or hear make us feel shameful, resentful, angry, or hurt? Or do we sense that something we said or did made someone else feel shameful, resentful, angry, or hurt? Sometimes awareness comes from others, from talking to those we know and trust. Talking to the right person (our sponsor, spouse, or boss, for instance) can give us perspective.

In Twelve Step recovery, awareness is noticing when our behavior is being driven by a character defect (such as dishonesty) rather than a spiritual principle (such as honesty). When we are aware of our behaviors and the motivations behind them (character defects or spiritual principles), we can make efforts to rectify a situation. We can also make a pretty accurate Tenth Step inventory and ask our Higher Power to remove these character defects so we can start the day with a clean slate.

Acceptance

Acceptance is the opposite of "self-will run riot." We accept people and situations as they are, not as we want them to be. We stop fighting what is and accept it as it is. We realize that what we're fighting is a universal force. We can't push against this force for long. Eventually, like addiction, it overpowers us and lays us flat out. When we accept things as they are, we go in the same direction as the universal force. We go with the flow.

At the very moment we do that, we've given our will over to our Higher Power so that it can create the best solution—not necessarily the solution we want or in the time frame we want, but the solution that is in the best interest for everyone, whether they see it that way or not. This is when events we might call miracles take place.

Right Action

Right action is acting from one or more of the Twelve Step principles: We act with honesty, not dishonesty; we act with justice, not unfairness; and so forth. Our actions are grounded in feelings of peace and serenity. Acting with integrity leaves us with an unmistakable feeling. We know we have done the right thing.

We don't necessarily need to ask our spouse or our best friend if we're doing the right thing. We know.

Right action isn't about being right or wrong. Sometimes we apologize even when we know we are "right," as far as the facts go. Sometimes it doesn't matter who's right. What matters is our behavior—how we respond, how we treat others, how well we handle our responsibility in a relationship. Sometimes right action is no action. It's patience.

— TAKEAWAYS —

» One day at a time means starting each day with a clean slate.

» Cleaning our slate requires the Tenth Step, prayer, meditation, awareness, acceptance, and right action.

» Recovery is a gift and requires that we live a balanced life.

» We raise our spiritual awareness when we live by the Twelve Step principles instead of by our character defects.

CHAPTER 9

RELAPSE (NOT AGAIN!)

"When you come to the edge of all you know, one of two things can happen: There will be something solid for you to step upon or you will learn how to fly."

—Author Unknown

PEOPLE ALWAYS FOUND it amusing that my young Italian mother, Toni, named her children Tom, Dick, and Harry. I was the altar boy, the Boy Scout, a tap dancer, and an attention getter. Dick, 5 years my senior, found his way into the James Dean culture of the 1950s. Dick drank with the "bad boys," also known as the "greasers." When I was 12 or 13, he gave me my first drink, a screwdriver, and my first cigarette. He was my hero. Dick died from this disease. I carry his ashes to every AA meeting I attend. He never did go to meetings like he was supposed to, so I just torture him in the afterlife.

Tom, 3 years my junior, is quieter, more introverted. Tom regularly drank vodka at lunchtime when he worked as a butcher. Someone told him 25 years ago that he didn't have to do that, and he stopped cold turkey. He never used a program of recovery. A few years ago, Tom stumbled out of his pickup truck, stone drunk for the first time in 25 years. This time he got into a program, and he's finally getting the idea that there's more to it than "just say no."

Relapse is the return of the signs and symptoms of addiction during recovery. It starts, most importantly, as a deterioration of recovery beliefs, behaviors, and attitudes and ends in the use of alcohol or drugs. Relapse is a process not an event, and using is the final stage in the process.

  Relapse is common. Although some people never relapse, others relapse repeatedly. Statistics regarding how and when recovering people relapse are unreliable usually because of denial. People are reluctant to admit to relapse when questioned in surveys, so the margin for error is large. We can safely state that 10 to 60 percent of people relapse usually in the first 6 months of recovery.

WHY WE RELAPSE

Relapse is common—but not inevitable—for several reasons, including post-acute withdrawal symptoms, stress, the fact that recovery programs are voluntary, and, most importantly, because it's easy to forget that addiction is a fatal disease.

Post-Acute Withdrawal

When we stop using drugs or alcohol, we enter into an acute withdrawal phase if the quantity and frequency of use was sufficient

MONITORING: A SAFE BET

The Federation of State Physician Health Programs' seminal Blueprint Study states that after 5 years, nearly 80 percent of physicians in 121 monitoring programs remained at work, sober, and without relapse for the entire 5-year period. That is an extraordinary result and attests to the fact that monitoring is much more than random urine testing for the use of an illicit drug or alcohol; it is a monitoring of a recovery process—the work environment, the work quality, and the principles of the program that have been incorporated into the life of the recovering physician.

All the patients in my recovery and wellness network are monitored after discharge from their level of care. The longer they are monitored, the better the outcome. Several outstanding monitoring organizations are now using this model for the layperson, providing these services to patients who wish to make it through the first or second year of recovery with that safety net built into their programs.

Monitoring is a safety net to be appreciated—not a punitive condemnation or sentence. *The purpose here is to comfort the disturbed and to disturb the comfortable.* And it's an opportunity to confront stubbornness, self-pity, and resentment.

enough to produce symptoms. Acute withdrawal symptoms, which can last 7 to 10 days, are mostly physical and vary depending on the person and the drug. But acute withdrawal symptoms are only the beginning of recovery. The mind may experience post-acute withdrawal symptoms that last for months after we stop using our drug of choice.

A condition known as post-acute withdrawal syndrome (PAWS)

affects us emotionally and mentally and can last for up to 2 years. Following are some common PAWS symptoms:

- An inability to think clearly

- Emotional overreacting (during good times or bad times)

- Memory impairment

- Problems sleeping

- Problems with physical coordination

- Stress sensitivity

After a head injury that results in a concussion, a person can experience post-concussion syndrome weeks to months later with exactly the same symptoms we see in post-acute withdrawal. Like a blow to the head, addiction damages its target, the brain.

Stress

Post-acute withdrawal symptoms and being in recovery can cause a lot of stress. Stress in recovery results from trying to cope with life's ups and downs without our chief coping mechanism prior to abstinence—without our drug of choice—all while suffering from lingering withdrawal symptoms.

The stressors don't even have to be bad. They may include milestones, anniversaries, vacations, changes in routine, boredom, or illness. All of the above can produce stress, and trying to cope with some degree of cognitive impairment simply worsens an already difficult situation. (About 70 to 90 percent of newcomers who arrive at a treatment facility may have demonstrable cognitive difficulties.)

A Never-Ending Process

Our recovery journey takes us well beyond withdrawal. It takes 2 to 3 years of sobriety to recover from the most serious biological problems brought on by our disease. And it takes 8 to 10 years to "normalize" into a sober lifestyle or to develop what we call emotional sobriety. We can work on our recovery daily for an entire decade before we feel "normal." The commitment required in recovery is a tall order even for the most earnest and diligent in our group.

Recovery Is Voluntary

Recovery is a voluntary, positive focus and growth toward a contented, productive life away from the addiction lifestyle. The term *addiction lifestyle* implies that addiction has a culture of its own—it has its own set of rules, customs, and values. Recovery also has a culture of its own with its own distinct characteristics. Because no one is chaining us to a recovery lifestyle, the option to quit is a matter of self-will. We can decide whether we want to stay in recovery or whether we want to return to the culture of addiction.

In a voluntary program, we have a choice to participate and are free to determine the extent and intensity of our participation. Abstinence may seem more possible with a gun to our head, but there is no gun in recovery. We must change ourselves.

If there is a metaphoric "gun" in recovery, it is the thought of a relapse. Relapse is more than a loss of recovery, beliefs, and habits. It is a biochemical event. When the brain perceives the chemical changes of stress, it directs us to engage in soothing behaviors, behaviors that will increase our levels of dopamine. Our brain is just doing its job—relieving our stress to achieve a state of homeostasis. Therefore, we must make an extra effort to voluntarily engage in our own recovery, knowing how easy it is for our body to slip back into dangerous behaviors.

A Fatal Disease

The disease of alcoholism and addiction is fatal and characterized by dependence, obsession, compulsion, and loss of control. It is always headed toward insanity and death. It is a chronic, organic disease of the brain with psychosocial consequences—it affects our thinking, our behaviors, and our relationships. It has a relapsing and remitting pattern and is treatable, one day at a time, but not curable; at least not as yet. It is genetically based, featuring symptoms of tolerance and withdrawal. Forgetting the fact that addiction is a fatal disease is often the first sign of relapse. In forgetting this important fact, we subtly adjust our approach to recovery in a take-it-or-leave-it fashion. Forgetting that it is a fatal disease means that, in our minds, there is far less at stake in persevering in a program of recovery.

THE ANATOMY OF A RELAPSE

Typically, in the anatomy of a relapse, a cascade of flowing events leads to that unfortunate drink or drug. It all seems to start with a change in the way we feel and a denial of those feelings—being dis-honest about those feelings. This leads to changes in mood, irritation, restlessness, annoyance, and anger. And soon we are starting to seek relief from the resentment, the self-pity, the frustration, the disap-pointment, and the sense of entitlement that we've endured as a result of those pent-up emotions. We shift the blame, tacking it on to others, and old friends and old haunts come back into focus in an aimless attempt to seek a solution.

I once relapsed in Europe, where, of course, my experience would not be full unless I drank a little wine. In this case, the change in feelings was from contentment to entitlement. And, because of my addicted brain, within a matter of hours, wine changed to brandy and brandy changed to grappa. The stronger the alcohol content, the better I liked it. Bingo. Twenty-four hours to a full-blown relapse.

On another occasion, I was taking a prescription legitimately given by my dentist. The prescription said to take one to two pills every 4 to 6 hours, but within 24 hours I was taking four to six pills every 1 to 2 hours. That wasn't what it said on the label, but it was what my body demanded. Bingo. Twenty-four hours to a full-blown relapse. Looking for more pills and unable to find them, I simply reverted back to my home base, alcohol, and there I was off and running again. I put myself in dangerous situations, trying to be abstinent in Club Med or on a cruise or with a bunch of friends at a football game, and the mood demanded to be satisfied. I was testing my newfound sobriety a little bit more than it needed to be tested, and "I'll just have one" would turn into "I just can't stop." The events in my life with similar outcomes are simply too numer-ous to mention.

The "committee" in our heads, the self-talk that convinces us to pick up a drink or drug again, is best characterized by structures that we now know to be in the limbic system. The limbic system is concerned with integrating all functions related to personal experience—memory, mood, learning, and emotions like sadness, anger, and fear. The limbic system is responsible for maintaining a healthy consciousness. If we are feeling uneasy, the limbic system triggers proteins in the brain that cause us to crave something that will bring us relief. If alcohol or drugs have given us relief in the past, we will want to turn to them for relief now. These "craving" proteins ensure the impulsivity, loss of inhibition, and compulsivity seen in relapse.

If relapse is a psychological and biological process in our brains that drives us toward spontaneous, dopamine-mediated actions that will bring us comfort, the cause of addiction is, arguably, stress and our reaction to it. Stress increases our requirements for dopamine, a neurotransmitter secreted by the midbrain in order to ensure repetitive survival behavior. It is not an option; it is a requirement of survival. As mentioned earlier, alcohol and drugs and their use can trump more appropriate survival behaviors, leading eventually to compulsive use with often fatal consequences.

The antidote for relapse is gratitude, dignity, humility, and self-respect.

WHAT IT MEANS TO TRIGGER ADDICTION

Certain circumstances, including sights, sounds, tastes, and smells, can trigger our senses and our memory banks to tap into the files in our past and recall those incidences where drugs were used to make us feel a certain way. Enormous happiness and elation, celebration, devastating sadness, isolation and loneliness, anger and exhaustion— these types of circumstances trigger our memory banks and put us in a state of stress. The triggered brain will then seek out the old drug, old behaviors, old friends, and old locations in search of that set of circumstances or substances that will relieve us.

Triggers can be very obvious—the sound of laughter from a bar, the smell of beer, the pop of a cork, the lighting of a pipe, the sight of a syringe, a beer commercial, an old song, a vacation, good news, bad news, an unexpected letter, enormous happiness, or enormous sorrow. Any of these can create the anxiety that triggers our brain to use.

ADDICTION IS ALWAYS WITH US

We are always recovering and never quite recovered. That is because as we get more time in sobriety, we become more aware of the enormous consequences of addiction. Its ability to resurface in our life becomes more, rather than less, evident. We can keep the disease in remission, but its capacity to resurface should never be underestimated.

When we think drinking or using is a logical choice because it is better than suicide or insanity, which seem to be the only other options, we're hard-pressed to come up with a reason not to relapse. Relapse is the process of being dysfunctional in sobriety. We paint ourselves into a corner; we convince ourselves using is logical; and we pick up our drink or drug—the end of the relapse process.

AM I ON TRACK?

If you can answer yes to the following questions, chances are you're on track with your Twelve Step recovery:

- Am I checking in with my sponsor daily?
- Am I going to meetings regularly?
- Am I seeing a therapist or counselor weekly?
- Am I reading recovery literature?

If you can answer yes to these questions, you may be relapsing and need to take action:

- Am I overly tired or frustrated?
- Am I telling white lies?
- Am I skipping meetings?
- Am I avoiding my sponsor?
- Am I using work or family responsibilities as an excuse for not working the program?

If we're not in a Twelve Step program, we can still relapse. The signs of an upcoming relapse may not involve missed meetings or avoiding our sponsor, but they are similar in many other ways. The principles that apply to each of the Twelve Steps are universal and serve as a good barometer for a relapse in progress. If you recall from Chapter 5, these principles include honesty, hope, faith, surrender, courage, integrity, willingness, humility, reflection, justice, vigilance, awareness, and service and charity. Being remiss about any of these principles can lead to behaviors that result in drinking or using again. Ideally, if those close to us tell us our behaviors are veering into relapse behaviors, we will want recovery bad enough to take action on our own behalf, perhaps by openly talking about our self-discoveries with family and professionals. We are looking for those signs of exhaustion and of weakening boundaries; of increased work schedules and decreased recovery schedules; of failure to keep promises and of little white lies—the subtle things that are often observed and not talked about.

SOME MYTHS ABOUT RELAPSE

Many people fear relapse and, as a result, have created a few myths along the way:

MYTH #1: Relapse is inevitable.

Relapse is common, but it's far from inevitable. About half of those who go through treatment relapse within the first year. About 30 percent of people who go through treatment are clean and sober in 5 years.

MYTH #2: Relapse means failure.

Relapse can be thought of as part of the process. Hopefully, we don't have to go through it. But, if we do, we haven't failed. We've given ourself the opportunity to see what part of our program wasn't working for us. We now know what we need to do this time to ensure we stay in recovery.

MYTH #3: Relapse can't be prevented.

Relapse is preventable. We must know the symptoms and make sure we're honest with our sponsor, friends, and family about our recovery. Others will point out the beginning of a relapse for us. If we listen, we can avoid a full-blown relapse.

MYTH #4: It takes years to hit bottom once you relapse.

Drinking or using even one time can bring our brain's reward system back to where it was when we last used. In other words, our body will crave the same amount of alcohol or drugs we were using when we quit. This can take a minute, a day, a week, a month, or a year. There's no way to predict how long it will take us to hit bottom.

MYTH #5: Relapse is necessary to strengthen one's recovery.

Relapse can show us what it is we need to focus on in our recovery program, but it's not necessary. We have sponsors, meetings, literature, our Higher Power, the Twelve Steps, and our spiritual awareness to strengthen recovery.

WHY BOTHER?

You may be wondering whether it's worth it. You might be thinking, *Why should I work so hard only to fail?* In recovery, relapse is not failure. When a person relapses, he learns a great deal about himself and his recovery program in a short period of time. He is able to identify his weak spots, the areas he needs to strengthen. Remember our earlier analogy to healing from a broken leg: Instead of getting only 80 or 90 percent better, in recovery a realistic goal is to improve 200 percent or more. Recovery is always worth the effort.

It is important to note that most relapses are unnecessary. If we can anticipate and identify the signs and symptoms, we can prevent relapse. Relapse starts with some lapse in sanity. When we realize that we are slipping into new ways of thinking and new behaviors that signal early relapse, where do we begin? We must be constantly vigilant, seeking second opinions from sponsors, friends, and family if we experience any of the red flags. The best way to do this is to make those close to us part of our relapse prevention plan.

YOUR RELAPSE PREVENTION PLAN

In recovery, it's essential to have a relapse prevention plan, or a set of automatic actions we and our family, boss, and counselor or therapist take should relapse start to rear its ugly head. This preordained set of actions clicks into effect if a urine test shows positive for alcohol or drug use or if someone observes relapse behaviors in us. We agree to the plan in advance—it is a signed contract.

A relapse prevention plan is always in writing. If we haven't gone through a treatment program, we can find templates for relapse prevention plans online or can order workbooks that help us process every aspect of relapse. We can talk to our sponsor about what his relapse prevention plan looks like and whether he's ever had to use it. When our sponsor knows us well enough, he can give us some input on what we might need to include in our personal plan. A relapse prevention plan is just as, if not more, important as any document we would keep in a home safe or in a safety deposit box. Making a plan requires our time and attention. We make it a priority in our lives.

RELAPSE RED FLAGS

The following thoughts and behaviors are all signs and symptoms of relapse:

- Argumentativeness
- Avoidance and defensiveness such as avoiding feedback and manipulating the meetings we go to (I'll only go to a speaker meeting—no one will call on me to offer my own opinions or speak of my feelings.)
- Blaming and loss of a constructive plan initiated by self-action (It's your fault!)
- Cockiness and complacency
- Confusion (I just don't get it.)
- Crisis building (Things are terrible; if only things were different.)
- Denial
- Depression (It's no use. I'm not sleeping well, and I'm not eating well. I'm actually thinking suicidal thoughts.)
- Dishonesty
- Elaborate excuse making
- Exhaustion
- Expecting too much from others and giving too little
- Feeling like your program has plateaued and is not progressing
- Forgetting gratitude
- Frustration
- Immobilization (Poor me.)

- Impatience
- Irresponsible rule breaking, recklessness
- Isolation (I feel trapped and hopeless.)
- Letting up on our own personal disciplines
- Loss of control (I'll go to fewer meetings, and I might as well use. I mean I'm not working my program. I might as well be out there drinking. Maybe that's what I'm supposed to be doing.)
- Neglecting personal appearance and hygiene
- Panic and anxiety
- Restlessness, irritability, discontentment
- Risk taking
- Self-pity (This is not going to get any better. I've lost my confidence. Maybe social drinking and social use of drugs is appropriate.)

- Switching poisons (I choose other addictive behaviors such as food, gambling, sex, or work.)
- Thinking it can't happen to me
- Thinking that I'm omnipotent
- Use of mood-altering chemicals (I can "slip" just this once. It won't hurt me.)
- Wanting too much from the program

And the most dangerous of them all . . .

- Option reduction (I feel trapped. I have feelings of insanity and suicide and think about using my drug of choice.)

Strategies

Our prevention plan includes statements that explain our strategy for staying clean and sober. Following are some ideas:

- I will remain abstinent from all mind-altering substances and behaviors.

- I will attend three to five or more Twelve Step meetings per week.

- If I don't have a sponsor, I will find a temporary sponsor immediately.

- By the end of 90 days, I will have selected a permanent sponsor.

- I will attend private or group therapy weekly with a certified relapse prevention counselor.

- If appropriate, I will go to family or couples counseling weekly.

- I will attend renewal workshops at least once every 6 months.

- I will inform my doctor and dentist that I am abstaining from mood-altering substances and should only be pre-scribed a mood-altering substance under the guidance of an addiction professional. Alternatively, I will find a doc-tor and dentist who are certified in addiction medicine.

- Each day, I will do a Tenth Step inventory and make amends when necessary to ensure my slate is clean. I will right my wrongs quickly.

People to Include

Because the first target of this disease seems to be our own personal awareness of how we are doing (we tend to think we are in far better shape than we are), outside opinions can be lifesaving. A relapse prevention plan involves many different people. The more people included in the plan, the better: family members, our sponsor, other AA/NA members, friends, our counselor or therapist, our physician, our employer, and, of course, ourselves. Like in an intervention, the people responsible for keeping tabs on us confront us with the evidence and remind us of the set of actions in our signed contract that are now going to take place.

Probably the most important part of a prevention plan is giving the people we put on the plan permission to approach us and give honest feedback spontaneously—at the very first sign that we are reverting back to old behaviors, attitudes, or actions or starting some new and unwelcome behaviors, attitudes, and actions. This is especially true for family members, the people we are sometimes the hardest on. Whether we realize it or not, our family is also in recovery. Our behavior has dramatically changed their behavior. What we do affects their recovery as well. We must give them permission to share or offer feedback regarding what they observe in our behavior.

A prevention plan is based on honesty, openness, and a willingness to subject ourselves to the accountability and feedback of the Fellowship. If we participate in Twelve Step meetings and sponsorship, we will be gifted with the early recognition of those changes that are often ignored, which are the earliest signs of relapse. The earlier they are discovered, the easier it will be to adjust our course and get back onto the path.

Common Actions and Consequences

Every prevention plan outlines actions we agree to take if we relapse. The deeper we are into our relapse, the more serious the actions and consequences. This portion of the plan keeps us honest and gives us and those involved immediate direction. Including a list of actions has the added benefit of consoling loved ones. When we give them a contract that lists constructive actions—consequences we agree in advance to face—they are much less likely to react with anger, mistrust, and panic if we do start to relapse. In the past, these reactions to our behaviors usually gave us an excuse to drink or use.

Actions and consequences usually include at least some of the following:

- 90 meetings in 90 days

- Daily contact with a sponsor

- Enrollment in an intensive outpatient program

- Moving to a halfway house (sober living house)

- A leave of absence from work to go to
  residential treatment

More serious consequences might include the following:

- Loss of professional licensure

- Jail time (if court-ordered to abstain for a period of time)

Follow-Up and Reinforcement

Constantly review and revisit your relapse prevention plan. Habit and structure equal freedom for the alcoholic or addict. The real work starts here: to protect the important investment we have made in ourselves.

THE AFTERMATH

I'd like to mention two important points about the emotional fallout of a full-blown relapse.

First, we must not beat ourselves up. This serves no good purpose and only adds to our shame. We are not the only people who've relapsed. The best course here is to take the next right action. We follow the actions outlined in our relapse prevention plan, and we start to feel better.

Second, part of the reason we might feel so inclined to beat ourselves up is that we've been moving forward, and have been geared up to move in that direction, and then we betray that mind-set. The result is often that drinking or using is not fun anymore. We now know too much, and to drink or use is to torture our good conscience.

— TAKEAWAYS —

» Relapse starts with a deterioration of recovery beliefs and behaviors. We can be relapsing even if we don't drink or use.

» A full-blown relapse is when we start drinking or using again.

» Relapse is common but not inevitable; relapses are unnecessary.

» A relapse prevention plan is a signed contract that involves many people.

» Relapse prevention plans include clear-cut steps we can take to get back on the recovery track.

» Others can usually see our relapse behaviors before we do.

» Relapse is not failure if we learn from our mistakes.

CHAPTER 10

UNDERSTANDING CROSS-ADDICTION

"Be yourself. Everyone else is already taken."

—OSCAR WILDE

ANDREW, A YOUNG physician, developed an addiction to opioid pain relievers. Because of his easy access to prescriptions and the inject-able forms of these drugs, his addiction escalated rapidly. By the time he entered treatment, he was in the throes of the disease with all of its most serious consequences: biological, psychological, social, and spiri-tual. His world had been shattered. But opioids weren't his only source of destruction.

Part of this disease is about entitlement, and this busy man abso-lutely felt entitled to relaxation, a healthy objective if sought in a healthy manner. Even though Andrew eventually abstained from opioids after receiving treatment, his sense of entitlement did not go away. Believing he deserved to feel good and relaxed by external means (as opposed to meditation, a connection with his Higher Power, and so forth), he began delving into behaviors that stimulated the dopamine system and gave pleasure in the absence of his drug of choice.

During Andrew's first 6 months of self-induced abstinence, he gained 60 pounds. He no longer used his drug of choice, so he turned to sweets (sugar), eating two or three desserts at a sitting. Soon, he tipped the scale at 280 pounds. When Andrew's cardiologist confronted him about his weight gain and urged him to lose weight, he began that diligent journey. Although he began to lose weight, his sense of entitlement still did not go away. The void that opioids, alcohol, and food once filled was once again reopened, and Andrew discovered the dopamine-releasing effects of the local gaming casino.

At first, he stuck with the slot machines. Isolated and absorbed in the machinery, he would escape into his own worry-free world. This, to him, provided the relaxation he felt entitled to. Like eating dessert alone in the kitchen, he could sit at one of these gambling machines and quietly anticipate the next card or the next big payoff. Andrew began spending more and more time and money at the casino, to the detriment of his relationships, health, and finances.

Dopamine is dopamine, whether it comes from substances in a glass, in pill form, or from varied behaviors. The hijacked addicted brain will respond in predictable fashion, creating an imbalance that can lead to enormous consequences.

In one simple sentence: Cross-addiction is the substitution of one mood-altering drug or behavior for another. Understanding cross-addiction is absolutely essential for the long-term success of the newly recovering individual. It is a trap that I've seen countless numbers of people fall into time and time again.

We get newly sober, finish treatment, and are on a roll in the Twelve Step program. We do our homework and find a sponsor and a home group, but we fall short in our vigilant awareness of a disease that is cunning, baffling, and powerful and that finds a way to come at us from any direction.

WHAT CROSS-ADDICTION LOOKS LIKE

There are many stories told of an alcoholic, newly sober, who goes to the dentist for much-needed dental work. It may not surprise you that dental problems are common because alcoholics and addicts are not always bastions of self-care and health maintenance. He goes and has some work done and gratefully accepts a prescription to help relieve the pain. The prescription is all too often an opioid such as Vicodin (hydrocodone with acetaminophen) or oxycodone. He takes the medicine as directed—one pill every 4 to 6 hours for pain. Soon he notices that pain relief is only part of the effect of the drug. He starts to realize that it actually feels good. He becomes a little euphoric or high. Immediately he experiences a craving, governed by chemicals in his addicted brain, and takes the next dose prior to the recommended time (perhaps in 2 or 3 hours instead of the recommended 4 or 6). Sometimes a physician or dentist gives the alcoholic or addict a "choice," as in, "Take one or two every 6 to 8 hours *as necessary* for pain." Well, an alcoholic or addict is going to take *two* every 6 or maybe every 4 hours. You get the picture.

The prescription runs out far sooner than intended. The addict calls the doctor and says, "My pain was more severe than I thought. I used up my medication. May I have another prescription?"

The doctor might write a prescription once or twice before saying, "I think you are using too much of this medication."

This is not a problem for a real alcoholic or addict. We'll simply go to another dentist or to the urgent care center, find someone else, and get a second prescription for the same medication. Before long, we have substituted our alcohol or drug with this new mood-altering chemical. It affects the brain in the same way our drug of choice does and, of course, affects our decision making, too. It is not long before we return to our drug of choice, figuring *I'm not a real alcoholic. I'm not a real addict. I'm not like those other people. I can handle it. Maybe I'll have just one.*

BEWARE OF LAME EXCUSES

The rooms in treatment centers around the world are filled with people who have fallen prey to cross-addiction: Valium (diazepam) or Xanax (alprazolam) for alcohol; muscle relaxants like Soma (carisoprodol) for heroin; marijuana for cocaine. Some end up addicted to lethal combinations. For example, the once-recovering alcoholic, newly addicted to Vicodin (hydrocodone with acetaminophen), begins to drink again. Soon he's taking both Vicodin and Valium or maybe also drinking alcohol at the same time. These lethal combinations often lead to unintentional overdose and death.

The thought process goes something like this: *Why is it harmful to just smoke a little pot? Why not just have a little glass of wine? I never seemed to have a problem with alcohol. My drug of choice was opioids.* We rationalize that it must be okay: *My doctor prescribed it. I didn't buy it off the street; I bought it at a drugstore.* In truth, we have simply been dishonest or failed to switch to a doctor or dentist who understands the disease of addiction and will protect our recovery at all costs.

These thoughts and lame excuses ultimately lead to disaster. The outcome is predictable: We trigger our addiction, this time to a new substance. It may happen instantly or it may take years, but eventually we acquire a whole new addiction or revert to our original drug of choice and present with a full-blown relapse.

A note to the very resistant patient: Those of you who rationalize continued drug or alcohol use despite having been diagnosed with a substance use disorder have not come to truly realize that addiction is a fatal disease. If you called your addiction "cancer," would you follow your plan?

ADDICTIVE BEHAVIORS

Certain addictive behaviors can alter mood just as powerfully as any drug. These behaviors, including over- or undereating or obsessive interest in sex, video games, the Internet, spending, gambling, and exercise, just to name a few, are also potential cross-addictions for the recovering alcoholic or addict. We need to be completely aware of our behaviors in recovery—and have a sponsor with whom we can be honest about those behaviors—so that we can immediately recognize imbalances in our lives that signal a leaning toward cross-addiction.

Why are some behaviors potentially addictive? They seem to

operate through the same mechanism as mood-altering chemicals: They affect that area of the brain where the desire to feel good all the time leads to repeating behaviors over and over in order to release natural mood-altering chemicals. It seems innocent enough, but eventually our judgment is affected, and we embark on that well-worn path back to our drug of choice.

NICOTINE AND OVER-THE-COUNTER DRUGS

Nicotine, one of the most powerfully addictive and damaging drugs of them all, enters the brain's neuropathways and stimulates dopamine. When used by the newly recovering individual, it decreases his or her chance for long-term sobriety by a very significant percentage. Because we now know the power nicotine has over recovering individuals, many treatment centers offer nicotine cessation programs to patients in treatment for alcohol or other drug addiction.

The concept of cross-addiction is extremely important even at Walmart, Walgreens, or Rite Aid. Over-the-counter medications can often lead to deadly relapses. We must be vigilant. "PM" medications like Tylenol PM (acetaminophen PM) and Advil PM (ibuprofen PM) contain diphenhydramine (Benadryl). Benadryl is a mood-altering medication that makes us feel relaxed and sleepy, as do NyQuil and Sominex, both used for sleep. Over-the-counter cough medicines and mouthwashes often contain huge amounts of alcohol, and when they're taken by the unsuspecting alcoholic or addict newly in recovery, the consequences can be disastrous.

A QUEST FOR WHOLENESS

Why do other substances and behaviors have such an effect on us? Although certain chemicals enter our brain's pleasure or, indeed, survival center via different pathways, they all seem to eventually come down the common pathway to stimulate the release of dopamine, the reinforcing chemical that tells us that our behaviors are necessary and need to be repeated in order for us to survive. If we've been down that road before, our pathways for addiction are hardwired and ready to reactivate. The alcohol or drug trumps other natural survival priorities. It becomes more important than nourishment, sex, relationships, and even breathing. We are held hostage by a brain with a broken and imbalanced reward system.

Dr. Carl Jung described the alcoholic or addict's craving for his drug of choice as a spiritual quest for wholeness. He observed that the alcoholic or addict is driven by a sense of incompleteness and emptiness that demands satisfaction. Dr. Jung knew that the addict's quest for wholeness would require some sort of spiritual solution as an alternative to the drugs and alcohol. Connected relationships based on honesty, identification, and accountability were where Dr. Jung felt the spiritual solution lies—not in other drugs or addictive behaviors.

Given that it is our nature to want to feel whole and that our brain's neural pathways have memory, we must be careful of cross-addictions. Just because a newly chosen chemical doesn't seem to resemble our drug of choice and enters through a different pathway doesn't mean that it won't trigger a relapse. Eventually it does the exact same thing that our drug of choice did, and it will bring us down.

PREVENTING CROSS-ADDICTION

Now that we know the substances and behaviors to avoid and understand what cross-addiction can do to our recovery, let's talk about how to prevent it from happening in the first place.

Include Cross-Addiction in a Relapse Prevention Plan

Preventing cross-addiction is preventing relapse. Addiction is addiction regardless of how we express it. We must be certain that our relapse prevention plan includes references to cross-addiction and that our family members, employer, and others are aware of the behaviors that constitute cross-addiction.

Talk about It

Remember that there is no greater preventive measure against the occurrence of relapse than to be absolutely honest with one's feelings and to be aware of any change in those feelings. In being honest, we communicate to someone we trust—usually a sponsor, a counselor, a family member, or other loved one—exactly how we feel. When we talk about it, it becomes real. When we talk about it, it becomes validated. Once we begin communicating, we may find that the most appropriate place to continue the dialogue is in a counselor's office or in a Twelve Step meeting room.

Have Ready Access to Contacts

We have to have ready access to sponsors and ready access to meetings. I keep a call list in my cell phone of about 10 close friends and sponsors. If I need to, I can go down the list, rapidly dialing numbers until someone picks up (and someone always picks up). I am never more than a minute or two away from an empathetic and sympathetic ear. I am able to discuss my problem so that it will be on the surface and will not go underground. I will not be ashamed of it, and it will not become a secret.

Give Others Permission to Give Feedback

It's vitally important to give family members and other loved ones permission to give us feedback should our behaviors cause them concern. We make it clear we will not punish them or get angry with them for sharing. The only consequence for sharing will be a thank-you. And why not? All they are doing is loving us.

Talk to Your Doctors

Have we discussed our addiction in the privacy of our doctor's or dentist's office? Have we told our doctors to put a notation in our medical chart indicating that we are intolerant of mood-altering chemicals? It's imperative that we be open and honest with the people who are in a position to prescribe mood-altering chemicals and who are responsible, to an extent, for our health. I can assure you that our doctors have heard the request before. We are, in all likelihood, not the only recovering addicts or alcoholics they treat. If they don't take us seriously, fire them and find someone who will.

Personally, I have had five surgeries while in recovery, each well planned with my anesthesiologist, my personal physician, my family, and my pain-management doctor. All pain medications were held by someone else and doled out to me as needed, so all pills were accounted for. No addiction issue has ever come from these surgeries, and substitutes used for pain relief did not put me in any danger.

Get in Touch with Your Addiction Professional

The American Society of Addiction Medicine (ASAM) is an association of physicians who are certified in addiction medicine or addiction psychiatry. They understand the disease of addiction and are familiar with cross-addiction and all issues associated with relapse. Visit their Web site at www.asam.org and use the "Find a Physician" feature to locate an addictions specialist in your area.

Quit Smoking

Smoking is a common substitute for other addictions, but it's a dangerous one. Research shows that people who quit smoking have a greater chance of staying clean and sober. For many, smoking is a trigger: Light a cigarette, pour a drink. Nicotine is a powerful drug and difficult to quit using. Get help by joining a quit-smoking program online or at your local hospital. The Centers for Disease Control and Prevention lists more than a dozen online or over-the-phone quit-smoking resources. Visit www.cdc.gov/tobacco/quit_smoking/how_to_quit/resources/index.htm for more information.

Carry a List of Over-the-Counter
Mood-Altering Medications

Ask your addictions specialist for a list of those over-the-counter medications that are dangerous. Laminate your list, carry it with you in your wallet, and refer to it often. It could save your life.

Below is a partial list of Class C drugs, which are generally safe to take, as they are not mood altering.

NASAL SPRAYS

Atrovent (ipratropium)

Ayr (saline)

HuMist (saline)

NasalCrom (cromolyn)

Ocean (saline)

COUGH/COLD/ALLERGY

Claritin

Robitussin guaifenesin syrup

Zicam Cold Remedy

ANALGESICS

Tylenol (acetaminophen)

NONSTEROIDAL ANTI-INFLAMMATORY DRUGS (NSAIDS)

Advil (ibuprofen)

Aleve (naproxen)

Motrin (ibuprofen)

ANTIHISTAMINES

Claritin (loratadine)

ANTITUSSIVES/EXPECTORANTS

Mucinex (guaifenesin)

GASTROINTESTINALS

Colace (docusate sodium)

Imodium (loperamide)

Kaopectate (bismuth subsalicylate)

Maalox (aluminum-magnesium antacid)

Mylanta (aluminum-magnesium antacid)

Pepcid (famotidine)

Pepto-Bismol (bismuth subsalicylate)

Prilosec (omeprazole)

Simethicone

Tums (calcium carbonate)

Zantac (ranitidine)

CHECK LABELS FOR THE FOLLOWING INGREDIENTS,

WHICH ARE NOT ALLOWED:

Dextromethorphan (DMX)

Diphenhydramine (Benadryl)

Pseudoephedrine

For more information on safe drugs, visit: www.dopl.utah.gov/programs/urap/forms/MedGuide.pdf

Be Familiar with
Mood-Altering Behaviors

If we know what behaviors release dopamine, we or those close to us can point out when we're starting to overdo it. We all need to eat, but we don't need to eat two desserts at a sitting. None of us needs to gamble or surf the Internet for hours at a time. When others point out that they believe we're going overboard on a mood-altering behavior, listen and get help.

— TAKEAWAYS —

» Cross-addiction is the substitution of one mood-altering drug or behavior for another.

» All mood-altering drugs (even if not our drug of choice) can lead to cross-addiction.

» Mood-altering behaviors include gambling, spending, over- or undereating, sex, and surfing the Internet.

» Like our drug of choice, cross-addictions release dopamine and fill a void.

» It's important to be honest with doctors and dentists about our addiction so they avoid prescribing us mood-altering prescription drugs or closely monitor us when these drugs are necessary.

» Cross-addiction is relapse and should be included on our relapse prevention plan.

CHAPTER 11

OPIOID AND PRESCRIPTION DRUG ABUSE

"But one led to two, two led to four, four led to eight, until at the end it was about 85 a day. The doctors could not believe I was taking that much. And that was just the Valium."

—COREY HAIM

AS A FRESHMAN in high school, Nick was diagnosed with ADHD by a guidance counselor. His parents followed up by taking him to a physician. Confident that the guidance counselor's diagnosis was correct, the physician didn't do any further testing to confirm the diagnosis. He reached for his prescription pad and wrote out a script for Adderall, which contains amphetamine, a stimulant. Nick had some behavioral problems as well, and over the course of his high school career, his doctor increased the dosage three times. By the time Nick entered college, he was on a fairly high dose of this mood-altering drug.

In college, the Adderall was like money. Nick would sell his medication to other students, leaving him without enough medication for himself, but he quickly learned how to manipulate the system. He started seeing three different doctors for his ADHD, and he obtained it on the Internet. He would then increase the dose to enhance his awareness and study capacity.

In addition, Nick told some friends to see their own doctors, after carefully coaching them on the symptoms they had to describe in order to get the diagnosis of ADHD, so they could get some similar stimulant drugs. There was no end to their manipulations: The dog ate my prescription; someone stole my pills; my car was robbed.

Similar stories are all too common, and the problem is probably not going away anytime soon, as the number of children diagnosed with ADHD continues to increase.

Nick's abuse eventually caught up with him. He went to treatment three times before putting together a year of solid recovery. He continues to work his program.

If you are addicted to prescription drugs, this chapter will give you some insight into how common (and dangerous) your drug of choice is. If you relapsed as a result of taking mood-altering drugs for pain, you'll learn your best next steps. If you are using any opioids—whether in the form of prescription painkillers such as OxyContin or street drugs, including heroin—you will learn that you are not alone.

If you are not addicted to prescription drugs, I encourage you to read this chapter to learn how pervasive prescription drug abuse is and how easily you could fall prey to it yourself—or even, unwittingly, be a source of these drugs for others.

A THREE-DECADE TREND

Prescription drug abuse is taking a medication "not as prescribed." Downing a few of Grandpa's painkillers to relieve a backache, a friend's Adderall to help get you through a night of studying, or a larger dose of your medication than the doctor indicated are all examples of prescription drug abuse. Although some people don't think anything of doing any of the above, these kinds of innocent actions are known to lead to bigger problems, as many of my patients will attest.

The statistics don't lie either. In 2009, 7 million Americans reported nonmedical use of prescription drugs—that was more than the combined number of people using cocaine, heroin, hallucinogens, or inhalants. By 2017, that number had increased to 18 million. In the three decades since the 1990s, about 870,000 people have died from prescription overdose in the United States. And the numbers have only recently shown signs of declining in a handful of states, mainly because of measures taken to help prevent opioid overdose deaths, which are of epidemic proportions in this country.

But the trend has gone on for far too long. Easy access to prescription drugs is part of the problem. Believing "it (addiction) will never happen to me" also contributes to the issue. Most people who enter treatment today are addicted to multiple drugs that often include medications taken for sleep, anxiety, ADHD, and obesity. The biggest culprit is painkillers, which fall under the umbrella of opioids.

OPIOIDS: A NATIONAL CRISIS

Prescription pain-relief medications, primarily opioids, are used in the United States more than anywhere else in the world. In 2018, overdose from synthetic opioids (opioid drugs made in a laboratory setting) made up two-thirds of all overdose deaths in the United States. Opioid addiction is an absolute national crisis.

The crisis started in the 1990s, when the medical community underwent a paradigm shift in treating chronic pain. Physicians were directed, as a matter of policy, to include pain as the fifth vital sign, along with blood pressure, temperature, pulse, and respiration. If you were hurting, physicians began to ask you to grade your pain on a scale of 1 to 10 or to pick out a smiley or sad face to indicate your pain level. In the decades just prior to this policy, the medical world was highly conservative when it came to doling out pain medications. They understood its potential for addiction. Yet many people were being undertreated for pain, and so the pendulum swung. This dramatic swing in the other direction was intensified by an atmosphere of direct-to-consumer advertising by the pharmaceutical industry.

Prescription painkiller addiction often leads people to do what they never thought they'd do: inject heroin. Heroin is cheaper than pills, and so gives users more bang for their buck. But it is in many ways more dangerous, given that it is often laced with fentanyl and other potent drugs. Using these concoctions can lead to a rapid and unexpected overdose as the drug inhibits the body's nervous system, specifically the breathing center. Reports of opioid overdoses have dominated the news and for the most part have steadily increased since the 1990s.

The opioid crisis shows little sign of waning. In 2018, nearly 68,000 people died from a drug overdose in the United States. Two-thirds of those deaths were caused by synthetic opioids. Synthetic opioids include prescription painkillers. According to the American Medical Association, most of the country saw increases in opioid overdoses in 2020, attributed in part to stressors associated with the COVID-19 pandemic.

Although opioid addiction is an ongoing problem in the United States and elsewhere, many other prescription drugs are also a source of concern when taken for too long or abused. These include many anxiety and sleep medications (depressants) and stimulants that are often prescribed for attention-deficit/hyperactivity disorder (ADHD), obesity, and narcolepsy.

The most significant long-term physical effects of prescription pills depend on the nature of the pills—whether they are stimulants or depressants. Unlike alcohol and methamphetamines, which have fairly predictable consequences from long-term exposure, prescription drugs seem to come to our attention more for accidents of chemistry—for the effects of lethal combinations. Overdose or lethal combinations lead to emergency department visits for cardiac arrhythmias, respiratory depression, cardiac arrests, and aspiration. (Aspiration occurs when the contents of the stomach are vomited up but the gag reflexes are so suppressed that the vomit ricochets off the top of the mouth and down into the lungs, causing infection or sepsis and oftentimes leading to shock and respiratory arrest.)

"PHARMING"

Billy's grandma got her hip replaced and was prescribed a number of painkillers and prescription medications. Being a tough old gal, she abstained from the pain medication in favor of a Tylenol and an icepack. Not wanting to be wasteful, she stored the painkillers in her medicine cabinet. A couple days later, she heard a knock at the door. It was Billy. "Hello, dear. I haven't seen you in ages! What are you doing here?" "Hi, Grandma! I'm just here to see how you're doin'! Make sure you don't trip or fall over any loose rugs! Hey, mind if I use your bathroom?" You can probably guess the rest. Billy searched through the medicine cabinet and grabbed some of Grandma's Restoril for sleep, Xanax for anxiety, and OxyContin for pain and stuffed the pills in his pocket. If Billy were to take those medications to a party, he might be guilty of "pharming," one of the scariest terms in addiction medicine today. Young people, usually ages 12 to 20, steal prescription medications, go to a party, and dump them into a large bowl. The pills are stirred up and consumed with alcohol. Someone reaches in and takes an unknown combination of Xanax and OxyContin or any number of lethal combinations. Some kids are fortunate and puke, while others wind up on the floor or in the emergency room. Drug abuse–related emergency room visits involving narcotics have risen dramatically since the mid-1990s, and the number of unintentional drug overdoses and deaths parallels the sale of prescription painkillers in the United States.

GETTING OFF PRESCRIPTION DRUGS

Mood-altering prescription drugs are powerful medicines that can produce some intense and dangerous withdrawal symptoms. Most withdrawal symptoms are drug specific. Withdrawal from amphetamines such as Adderall, for instance, constitutes a physical and psychological crash. Patients experience major depression and a desire to isolate. Devoid of hope, they need long hours of bed rest and support in the form of therapy. There are a few medications used for the detoxification. Withdrawal from benzodiazepines (such as Valium, Xanax, and Ativan) and the "Z" drugs (Ambien, Lunesta, and Sonata, to name a few) can be similar to withdrawal from alcohol in that it can be deadly. These drugs have a withdrawal syndrome that is marked by great excitation in the body and all the symptoms that go along with that, including sweating, rapid heartbeat, high blood pressure, extremely severe anxiety, and insomnia.

The danger of having seizures during withdrawal from opioid medications is great, and medically assisted detoxification is absolutely imperative. Medically assisted detoxification spares us from the inordinate suffering found in the old cold-turkey scenario. (The term cold turkey comes from the goose-bump flesh that many encounter in an opioid crash.) Other common opioid withdrawal symptoms include tearing eyes, runny nose, profuse sweating, profound anxiety, diarrhea, and deep, full-body pain often described as bone pain. In medically assisted detoxification, most of these symptoms can be relieved by medications, blood pressure can be lowered easily, and the patient can be gently let down from the high doses of opioids that he or she has been taking.

If you have tried to stop taking prescription drugs and felt these incredible flu-like symptoms, forcing you to restart your drug of choice to relieve your discomfort, take advantage of a medically supervised detoxification before attempting to abstain again.

HOW TO AVOID ABUSING PRESCRIPTION DRUGS

You can take several simple precautions to avoid getting involved with prescription drug abuse—whether for the first time, as a cross-addiction, or as an unwilling participant in another's addiction.

Be Knowledgeable

Know what your physician is prescribing. Ask whether the medication is mood altering.

The most commonly abused prescription drugs are opioids, depressants, and stimulants. Be aware, too, that some over-the-counter drugs can be equally addictive.

Opioids: Opioids include morphine, opium, hydrocodone, codeine, fentanyl, and heroin. Opioids produce a relaxed feeling in most people and are prescribed to relieve pain. Common brand names include OxyContin, Vicodin, Percocet, and Tylenol with codeine.

Depressants: Depressants "depress" the central nervous system and are therefore known as downers. They include alcohol, barbiturates, and benzodiazepines. Benzodiazepines such as Valium, Xanax, and Ativan and their close cousins, the "Z" drugs (Ambien, Lunesta, and Sonata), may be prescribed as a sleep aid or to relieve anxiety. GHB, one of the "date rape" drugs, is prescribed for narcolepsy but is abused by some bodybuilders.

Stimulants: Stimulants include amphetamines and cocaine. Ritalin is a common amphetamine prescribed for ADHD. Students, sometimes encouraged by parents, may take it as a study aid because it keeps them awake for hours. Ritalin is swapped among college students like jelly beans. Nicotine, methamphetamine, Ecstasy, bath salts, and "Smiles" are also stimulants.

Be Clever

Refuse a prescription for 30 Vicodin (hydrocodone with acetaminophen) after dental surgery. Ask for three pills instead. If you need more, you can get them, but three or four should get you through the first couple of days without risking the chance that you're going to become dependent and have to detoxify from these medications, whether you are an addict or not.

Be Wise

Be a wise consumer and recognize that medications need to be properly disposed of rather than stored in a medicine cabinet where young hands may seek them (or where you might be tempted to find them for yourself). There are many weapons of mass distraction—and destruction. I am particularly sad to see that my beloved profession and its prescription pad may have become one of them.

— TAKEAWAYS —

» Prescription drug abuse is so widespread it's a national crisis.

» The opioid crisis has for the most part steadily increased since the 1990s.

» Emergency room visits are common for people who take lethal combinations of prescription drugs or too much of a single drug.

» Cardiac arrest and aspiration are some causes of death due to prescription drug abuse.

» Withdrawal symptoms can be intense. A medically supervised detox is imperative.

» Withdrawal symptoms can be intense. A medically supervised detox is imperative.

CHAPTER 12

HOPE SURVIVES

"Even if you are on the right track, you'll get run over if you just sit there!"

—WILL ROGERS

MARIE, A 19-YEAR-OLD and a mother of a 3-year-old, first entered treatment without enormous consequence in her life. Her drugs of choice were alcohol and marijuana. Having a father in law enforcement, Marie felt she was coerced into getting help. She didn't necessarily want it. The young adult program she was in was designed to be a minimum of 90 days and to direct her toward a sober college experience, but after 30 days she had just had enough.

Her shame worked on her in many ways: She felt judged for becoming a mother at the age of 16, judged for her lack of maternal instincts, judged for her dependence on her mother for help in caring for her child. She felt judged for her socioeconomic status and even for the clothing she wore and her hygiene practices. In essence, she was her own worst judge. Marie, a very sweet girl, was accepted lovingly by her group and peers but could not let up on the shame that plagued her to the point where she felt she didn't even belong on the earth. Indeed, the disease of addiction used this much to its advantage, because after 30 days, she felt she needed a reward for that period of abstinence. She left treatment with some degree of obstinacy and against all professional advice. Her celebration included a drug she had never tried before: heroin.

Marie's addiction worked overtime to prove to Marie that her feelings of worthlessness were real. Within a year, she went from snorting heroin to injecting 4 to 5 grams a day. She shared dirty needles, had multiple sex partners, and mixed her drug of choice with huge doses of Xanax and occasionally methamphetamines. She was living on the streets, moving from Dumpster to Dumpster.

Marie begged her father to take her back to treatment, where she had once felt accepted. Now at 20 years old, she looked more like 39. Her clothes were dirty, her body was soiled, and her teeth showed signs of neglect. But despite all this, I remember the sparkle that appeared in her eye when I told her that she was just sick—that she was worthy of treatment that would make her well and able to take care of her child.

That sparkle was proof positive that no matter how far down our addiction takes us, hope survives. And as long as we have hope, we can recover.

We've covered a lot of information in this book, some of which is likely new and possibly overwhelming at first. But when we look at the program as a whole, it's really quite simple. A paragraph in the basic text of the Big Book sums it up quite nicely:

> Abandon yourself to God as you understand God. Admit your faults to Him and to your fellows. Clear away the wreckage of your past. Give freely of what you find and join us. We shall be with you in the Fellowship of the Spirit, and you will surely meet some of us as you trudge the Road of Happy Destiny. May God bless you and keep you—until then.

Let's review some of the most important concepts of recovery.

AWARENESS AND ACCEPTANCE

To stay in recovery 24/7, we need to fully accept that we need to be aware of our thinking and behavior 24/7. If we don't have conscious contact with our sponsor on a regular basis, if we don't have people in our life whom we can turn to when we need help, we'll get up in the morning, get dressed for the day, stand in front of a mirror, and say, "I'm okay."

We always need a second opinion. Most of us won't even have an idea that relapse is happening until someone hits us over the head or we have a drink in our hand. That's how most of us get to a full-blown relapse. Maybe you can relate to the cycle of waking up in the morning with that hangover, forgetting whom you may have called or hung out with the previous night, then making a few phone inquiries, talking around it until someone gives you a clue or two. The disease of addiction overwhelms my imagination with its longevity. It's been around forever, and I've never seen anyone who could beat it. Not anyone who has the genetic makeup for it. Beating addiction— or using without loss of control—is an absolute impossibility, and it always has time on its side.

BALANCE: ONE DAY AT A TIME

In the program, we learn that now means *now*. It is the only time that we have some semblance of any control in our life, and even *that's* on loan. Each day, we spend 90 percent of our energy on today (on the "now"), 5 percent honoring our heritage and our past, and the remaining 5 percent trying to do some appropriate planning for the future. But if we change those percentages, we fall into imbalance and are rocked right to our shoes. We get into our head and out of the present. We reverse the Third Step—my will, not Thy will—and we're off and running in the wrong direction.

Although I and countless other addicts live with the potential for imbalance every day, I don't worry about it constantly. It seems to be taken care of for me in one simple exercise: Each morning, I roll over onto my stomach, and before I hit the bathroom, I slide out of bed onto my knees and recite my interpretation of Steps One, Two, and Three: "There is a power that wants to kill me, and there is a power that wants me to live. Do I want to live or die today?" I do this every morning. Then, I start my day and maybe find another alcoholic or addict who needs some help or who will help me.

The purpose of a one-day-at-a-time approach to the disease of chemical dependency is to make the solution possible and to achieve success since control of addiction is impossible. We have the opportunity for salvation, one day at a time, even in the earliest phases of our recovery. We get a glimpse of hope and the will to move on, to move toward the light, to realize that the promises of this program have yet to unfold before us gradually, one day at a time. We get the benefits very early, and they expand. We don't have to wait to achieve long-term sobriety before we see the first hint of a promise come true in our lives. The simple relief, the daily reprieve from the obsession to drink or to use, is a promise in and of itself, realized in the first hour or day after someone has committed to abstinence. It is a *be-here-now* philosophy, necessary when we are trying to convince people to do something that they are persistently and vigorously disinclined to do—stop using.

I like to think of one day at a time as a way of coaxing the desperate and forlorn into a philosophy of hope that is needed for spiritual transformation. The Twelve Step meeting is the basic building block of this program, and it involves true involvement and participation. We need to attend these meetings early on, one or two daily, so that we can begin to weave the principles of the Twelve Step program into our lives, both in and out of the meetings.

I love to consult with my Vermont sponsor, the one who runs a pizza shop. He's a very nuts-and-bolts kind of guy with a gift for simple wisdom. I asked, "Would you think about how one day at a time works for you? I want to include it in a chapter I'm working on." In his inimitable fashion he said, "Well, I'm going to need to get back to you in a week or so on that." About 10 days later, I called him back. We had a nice conversation. He asked how I was, how my son was, and how my wife was. He asked how my program was going and what step I was working. And then he said, "By the way, I've been thinking about that one-day-at-a-time question you asked."

"Yes," I replied, anxiously awaiting his response.

He simply said, "For me, one day at a time means I just don't get overwhelmed." There you have it. One day at a time is an adopted attitude for a group of people who are desperate and impatient. The specter of a life without that best friend—alcohol or drugs—of having to cope with problems without that best problem solver—alcohol or drugs—is an ominous prospect. But if we don't bite off more than we can chew, we realize that recovery is probably something we can do at first for one minute, then for one hour, then for one morning, then for one day at a time.

We must keep it simple. We find the safety we need to be able to share and to identify. We are exposed to new friends in the Twelve Step meeting and get a bird's-eye view of what a sober life can be like, definitely not all roses but certainly manageable. We learn the tools of our program and how they get us from one moment of desperation to the next moment of faith and hope. We learn that the tools to transform our spiritual focus from the culture of addiction to the culture of recovery are given to us if we ask for help each day. These are the tools that will help us begin our spiritual quest, moving from fear to trust, from self-pity to gratitude, from resentment to acceptance, and from dishonesty to honesty. We move on from a precontemplative phase and are ready to change. Saying "I'll do it tomorrow, I'm not ready now" is a thing of the past, and today we can say, "Okay, I'll give it one day. That's all. I'll give it one day, and if I like what happens by the end of the day, I may decide to do it again tomorrow."

Remember: If we qualify for the disease of alcohol or drug dependence, we probably have some reasonable degree of thinking impairment, i.e., cognitive dysfunction. It affects our ability to solve problems. We may dwell on the past and feel guilt or shame over those events. We may feel anger, resentment, or doubt. We may become weak, hopeless, arrogant, and distracted. We may resort to blaming and denial and become stubborn—harboring doubt, grief, and self-pity. Jealousy, fear, panic, and relapse behavior may enter our lives, and we may engage in dangerous activities involving selfishness, gossip, and lying. We may become more self-centered, isolated, and lazy. There is still a lot of wreckage in our past that can affect a clean and pure moment today if we choose to visit it. The goal of this program is to *not* put more on our plate today than we can handle. As my Vermont sponsor says, "Don't get overwhelmed." Our Higher Power provides for us in a way that keeps our plate from overflowing if we don't inject our will to take on more than we can handle.

The negative feelings and behaviors that stem from cognitive dysfunction, combined with the character defects that the chemically dependent person possesses, can result in an imbalance at any point in time. These are the telltale signs that our lifestyle is becoming vulnerable to relapse. Stress and anxiety, restlessness, irritability, and discontent may need to be relieved. We now know that certain chemicals in the brain cause cravings to prompt us to relieve stress. Our brain remembers those substances that gave us relief in the past, and we will try to seek them out through old haunts, old friends, and euphoric recall. We get involved in a return of our denial and obsessive thinking. The result usually ends with some bad decisions. If we participate in unsafe behaviors, we are back to seeking and/or using our drug of choice before we know it. As I stated in Chapter 9, just *thinking* in this fashion, even without using, is relapse.

THE CLEAN SLATE

I can't say enough about the vital role that a Tenth Step takes in a day in the life of the alcoholic or addict. It gives us the opportunity to take personal inventory and, when we are wrong, to promptly admit our mistakes. We can clean our slate once, twice, even three times a day—going over our morning, finding out where we might have strayed, whom we might have offended, and making things right without carrying that burden into the afternoon. We can do it again at suppertime and once more at bedtime. If we go to sleep with a clean slate—our *i*'s dotted and our *t*'s crossed—we will wake up with a clean slate.

We know, as alcoholics or addicts, that we are powerless over our drug of choice. We know that our lives have become unmanageable, that there is hope and a power that wants us to live, and that we must decide we want to live enough to turn our will over to it. There you have it. Even before we've made it to the bathroom upon awakening, we've taken the first three steps each day.

Our first duty when we get on our knees in the morning is to thank our Higher Power for the grace bestowed on us and to ask for help this day to live life with dignity and the knowledge of His will for us. We ask for strength to act in accordance with that will.

STRUCTURE

Addicts and alcoholics need structure. The AA program and the programs we offer at the Betty Ford Center are structured, and success lies in the *doing* of it—not just living it, not just knowing or studying it. We define our personal behaviors and are aware of them so that early on we are able to catch ourselves straying from the path. Recovery is a voluntary, positive focus on—and growth toward—a contented, productive life away from the addiction lifestyle. That means we are walking the walk and our house is in order. We are checking our motives and our alternative agendas to be certain we are pure of heart this day.

The work we must do, one day at a time, is designed for recovery enhancement. We are depositing recovery capital into our bank account each day to be drawn upon during times of stress, crisis, or need. We deposit a positive attitude, right actions, acceptance, awareness, surrender, and connection with others. We deposit new spiritual focus. We deposit our ability to listen, to discover, to protect ourselves, to tolerate others, and to practice patience. We deposit our achievements, our willingness to survive, our appreciation, and our accountability. We deposit our service, our gratitude, and our survival. What we get from this work is a sense of emotional sobriety.

We are connected spiritually to a recovery program through sponsorship and relationships mutually based on the desire and the need to be sober. We act in congruence, doing good both for ourselves and for the world in which we live. The result is gratitude, dignity, and self-respect. So, in thinking about the next 24 hours, we don't have to struggle; we can relax and take it easy. We can ask for direction. One. Day. At. A. Time.

CHAPTER 13

MAKING THE FIRST MOVE

"Whatever you can do, or dream you can, begin it.
Boldness has genius, power, and magic in it."

—GOETHE

PROCRASTINATION IS NO stranger to me. I knew as a teenager that I drank like my father—that is, not normally but alcoholically. I'd have at least one or two drinks just to get over the paranoia that my next episode of alcohol intake would mean that I was becoming an alcoholic, just like my father. I pushed that notion off time and time and time again. As early as 1978, I was going to my first Twelve Step meetings. But I kept taking back my power, kept attempting to control alcohol and drink normally. Beginning in 1983, I enjoyed 5 years of abstinence but no recovery. Again, I was just putting off the inevitable, thinking that stopping alone, white-knuckling it without any program, would keep me sober. But it did much more. It created in me a sense of anxiety, longing, and sacrifice that could only end in a drink. It was just a matter of time.

It can be difficult to know when you're *ready* for treatment. But it's a no-brainer to know that you need to interrupt this disease of addiction. If you are under 21 and drinking or using illegal drugs, that's a hint that things are out of balance for you. It doesn't necessarily mean you're addicted, but it's worth the effort to take a good hard look at your behaviors. If you're preoccupied with thoughts of when you can smoke your next joint or pour the next drink, you might have a problem. If you are secretly getting prescription medications from more than one doctor, repeatedly taking more pills than recommended, or using for the effect rather than for therapeutic reasons, it's probably time to take a closer look at the relationship between you and your drug of choice.

REVELATION

The following conversation transpired between my son, Aram, and me when he was about 7 months into his own recovery.

Aram, with whom I thought I had been an extraordinarily present father, announced to me that he and my nephew had been stealing drugs out of my medicine cabinet and my home office for years and trading them for alcohol. I asked, "Did you trade it for pot?"

"No, we just smoked yours."

"My God! How did you get through high school?"

"High school? Dad, I was 11."

His answer shocked and rattled me, and I was suddenly in the presence of my disease and just how profoundly it permeated my life and all of my roles.

So what's your first move? Well, picking up and reading this book was certainly a terrific first step in the right direction. The more you understand the dead end of addiction and the hope that recovery brings, the more likely you will be willing to accept help for this disease. The concepts outlined in this book will hopefully support you in your efforts to find peace and serenity. Maybe this book or others like it are all you need to begin your recovery journey. But most people benefit from having some assistance, certainly in the form of AA or NA meetings and often in the form of inpatient or outpatient treatment. The power of a single phrase from a counselor or a story told by another addict in group can give you the "aha" moment that might otherwise take years to come. There's no shame in going to treatment for alcohol or drug addiction—only compassion and support. And treatment centers across the nation are set up to provide you with expert help.

You might know someone who has managed to stay clean and sober by quitting cold turkey and attending AA or NA meetings. On the other end of the spectrum is the individual who's been in every inpatient treatment program across the country—multiple interventions, multiple treatments, and multiple relapses. Every person and every situation is unique.

Volumes have been written about how to know when someone is ready to accept help, how to go about getting him or her help, and how to determine which treatments are necessary. Let me try to keep this as simple as possible: How you go about getting into recovery is unique to you. Recommendations for inpatient treatment, outpatient treatment, extended care, halfway houses, or AA or NA meetings should be individualized. Everyone's situation is different, and everyone's case is complicated by different

(continued on page 206)

WORDS OF ENCOURAGEMENT

The following letter, written by an unknown author, has inspired many new to recovery.

Letter to a Newcomer in AA

Congratulations! You may have taken the biggest step since Neil Armstrong stepped on the moon. Please note I said "may have." What you have done is given yourself the opportunity to make some choices, and you do have choices to make.

Having hit bottom myself, I would not be at all surprised that your brain is thinking more negative emotions than exist, including but not limited to fear, anger, remorse, resentment, and self-pity. I certainly hope they are doing a number on you. They will subside and go away, but they should *never* be forgotten. Keeping them in your memory will be a most useful tool for understanding yourself and for understanding others you may someday be in a position to help.

Actually, alcohol, in and of itself, was never my problem. Let's face it, the vast majority of people who drink alcohol never have a problem with it. For me, it was available to me in my teenage years, so I took it, not knowing it would eventually lead me straight to hell. Other drugs just were not available to me at that time, and if they had been, I probably would have dived into those, too. My real problem centered in my mind. I didn't know it then. For reasons unknown to me at the time, I was suffering from an incurable disease I had had since childhood. Alcohol did for me what it does for all of us alcoholics: It immediately set in motion a lifestyle that included drinking as an almost natural part of our lives, which, once begun, eventually turns into an intense craving for more and more.

Some of us manage to find our way into the Fellowship of

Alcoholics Anonymous through varied avenues—treatment centers, a nudge from the judge, the recommendation of our doctor or a therapist, a mandate from a parole officer—or, after hitting the bottom of the slime bucket, we manage to crawl into the program ourselves out of sheer desperation. And once begun, we learn how to keep our disease in remission one day at a time. Those few of us who manage to do what is suggested become stronger and happier than even our nondependent counterparts. But all that is a lifetime process of recovery that takes time, effort, and patience. The rewards are fantastic, believe me.

That process of recovery can be either a painful, miserable experience to be begrudgingly endured or it can be one of enlightenment, revelation, and joy. It's a choice you need to make. It involves honesty, open-mindedness, and willingness. Sounds like an easy choice to make, but you would be astounded at the large percentage of people who choose the pain and the misery because they don't want to get out of the driver's seat, want to hang on to their character defects and give lip service to honesty, open-mindedness, and willingness.

I always thought I was above average in intelligence, and maybe you think you are, too. At the very least, I thought I was a lot smarter than some of those clowns who were giving me suggestions. They kept it simple because they were simple-minded people (I thought). I kept it complicated by being convinced I was a lot smarter and knew all the answers until someone told me to take the cotton out of my ears and shove it in my mouth. They told me my very best thinking is what got me into the slime bucket to begin with. After that I began to listen—and the revelation began!

This was intended to be a morale booster, not a lecture. Sorry

(continued)

WORDS OF ENCOURAGEMENT *(CONT.)*

about that, but not really. I am so hung up on the wonders of recovery, I get carried away. What amazes me is what I have learned and the changes that have taken place in my life over the years. Each year I think it just can't get any better, but it does.

If you can get your butt out of the driver's seat; get brutally honest with yourself; erase all opinions, ideas, notions, and conceptions (more than likely, this is impossible, but it's something to shoot for); and become totally willing to take whatever steps are necessary to recover, the second half of your life can be filled with happiness you never dreamed possible. It has happened to me, and it has happened to millions, I mean millions, of others.

I am rooting for you because I care and I know and have experienced the absolute wonders of recovery.

Sincerely,
Anonymous

factors: relationships, finances, mental health issues such as depression, and medical consequences. The list goes on and on.

Hopefully you have taken the questionnaire on page 25 of this book to determine whether you need help. But if you think you have a problem, you probably have a problem. If someone's telling you they're worried about you, you're probably worth worrying about. If you've fallen down, ruined your car, ruined your suit, embarrassed yourself at a party, forgotten what you said on the telephone, gotten a discerning eye from your employer—what are you waiting for? It can only get worse. That's guaranteed. Is that what you're waiting for?

The fact that you have this disease is not your fault. It's not about morals or values or self-will. You're not a bad person; you are most likely a good person who has a very bad, even fatal, disease. If you respect yourself and those around you, it's your responsibility to get some help.

If you are the type of person to ignore a nasty-looking mole on your arm, in a sun-exposed area, that is morphing each day into something larger and more irregular, I don't know that I'm going to get through to you. But if you want to live—and I hope you do—now's the time to ask for help. There are a hundred different ways to seek help for the disease of addiction. Here are a few of the most common routes.

TALK TO A FRIEND

Talk to a friend who's in recovery or a trusted friend who knows someone in recovery. You might be surprised at how easy it is to find someone in recovery (there are millions of us). Arrange to just talk about what you're going through. Initial baby steps like this are important. They can set the whole thing in motion.

GO TO A TWELVE STEP MEETING

If treatment looks appropriate, the cheapest route is Alcoholics Anonymous. Go to an open meeting with a friend and just listen for the first time. You may need more—preferably, your needs should be determined by an evaluation—but going to a meeting is the best way to get your feet wet. Keep in mind that you may need a medically assisted detoxification. In some cases, detoxification without medication can be deadly.

ENTER OUTPATIENT TREATMENT

If you're lucky and the disease hasn't entwined you and your life to a great extent, a simple outpatient program may be perfect. Outpatient treatment gives you the flexibility to continue going to work or school. In addition, some insurance companies require that you first go through outpatient treatment before they'll approve you for residential care. You'll want to engage in outpatient treatment for at least 8 to 12 weeks with trusted, loving professionals. You'll want to monitor the disease after treatment. Treatment is a change in attitude, a change in lifestyle, and a change from the culture of addiction to the culture of recovery—a change that requires nurturing and daily maintenance. We can liken it to committing to a workout plan. The results start slowly and then become remarkable, but they do have to be maintained.

SCHEDULE A CLINICAL DIAGNOSTIC EVALUATION

The Rolls-Royce in the process for getting help with addiction is called the Clinical Diagnostic Evaluation. If you are not sure whether you have the disease of addiction, if you and your family are in doubt but you continue to be plagued by the unpredictability of your use of drugs or alcohol, this evaluation can save your life. Working over 4 to 5 days, a team of experts takes your history, gives you a physical examination, a psychosocial examination, a psychiatric examination, a full psychological evaluation, and psychometric testing. They use forensic evidence—body fluids, hair and nail analysis—to determine the level of use based on facts, not memory. They assess the quality of your relationships. They speak with friends and colleagues you give them permission to speak to and ask them what the impact of drugs and alcohol has been in your life.

Many of the patients I work with require solid evidence of their addiction. A thorough evaluation provides that evidence. It often reveals a previously overlooked mental health issue or trauma that contributes to drug use. Interestingly, more and more we are able to link drug use to what's known as transgenerational trauma. In these cases, the children or grandchildren of people who endured a trauma experience similar symptoms, including nightmares, anxiety, and fear. They carry the memory across generations, even when details of the trauma were never discussed with them.

Many people who suffer from trauma or mental health issues will self-medicate with alcohol and other drugs. So it's very common to see addiction in the aftermath of a traumatic event or as a result of depression or other mental health issues. A thorough evaluation pinpoints the issue by dotting all *i*'s and crossing all *t*'s. The revelations are often a relief to patients.

When the team of experts is done with the evaluation, they pass their recommendations on to you, your family, and any other parties you've agreed to share the information with. What you do with the results is up to you.

Not everyone who comes in for an evaluation is diagnosed with addiction or given treatment recommendations. If the diagnosis is addiction, it's hard to avoid the truth when it's right there in black and white. But the most important thing is that you've taken this monumental step.

THE ROCK-BOTTOM MYTH

Hitting rock bottom is not required before you seek help. In fact it's preferable that your bottom be higher than most. That is why I've written this book and that is why the millions of people who've been through this already are extending a hand, trying to save you from further and deeper pain and suffering.

Waitstaff in Mexican restaurants sometimes bring out fajitas on a sizzling hot plate. One waiter clears a path through the crowd, and the other one is dressed with large heat-resistant mitts, arms outstretched, holding a smoking and sizzling platter. When he sets it down in front of you, you lean back away from the heat, sweat dripping off your brow. The waiter kindly suggests, "Please don't touch the plate—it's very hot!" If you're like me, as soon as the waiter turns around, you stick one little finger on the edge of the plate. *How hot is it? Enough to hurt my finger? It can't be that hot. What is he talking about?*

Treating addiction before you hit rock bottom is kind of like preventing you from having to experiment with catastrophe, keeping you from having to relive the pain and consequences of the thousands of people who tell these stories every day. It's that simple. Don't touch the hot plate. It's not necessary, and it's not worth it. Take the advice. Intervene now and see the miracles happen in your life.

So if you even just think you have a problem, take the first baby step, the move that gets everything in motion, the move that gets you unstuck and that gives you relief. It's one step in the right direction, and it's easier than you think.

EXCUSES

Addiction hijacks the brain and, along with it, some of our good sense. Chances are high that, for every good reason you come up with to get help or to confirm whether you need help, you'll have reasons (i.e., excuses) why it won't work for you at this moment in time. That's your addiction talking. Learn to recognize when you're kidding yourself. Every time you say no to recovery, think hard about what's at stake. Is the world going to end because you might need to take a leave of absence from work? Is your child going to be permanently scarred because you need to focus more on yourself right now? Is your wife going to leave you for trying to get help and improve your marriage? Is your place of worship going to shun you for not being there every week? The effect of recovery is that your employer, your co-workers, your child, your spouse, your priest, pastor, or rabbi are going to benefit from you being the principled person you become in recovery. The truth is, there's no excuse for continuing down the road of destruction and bringing everyone in your path down with you.

Having said that, you will still make excuses, sometimes 50 layers deep. Because they seem to come from a bottomless pit, I'm going to give you a few dozen very simple ways to start the ball rolling.

- Ask people close to you if they think you might have a problem.

- Call a help hotline (you can be anonymous).

- Call a local treatment center to schedule an assessment.

- Call someone who's in recovery.

- Visit www.bettyfordcenter.org for contact info or to chat with someone online.

- Call your insurance company to see if chemical dependency treatment is covered.

- Call your local AA or NA chapter (look up the number in the Yellow Pages or online).

- Check out an AA or NA meeting.

- Check with your local hospital about their detox program.

- Google "addiction help."

- Google "addictions counselor" and your town.

- Imagine how your friends and family will describe you at your funeral.

- Confide in someone supportive.

- Imagine life 10 years from now if you are the best you can be.

- Imagine life 10 years from now if you keep drinking or using.

- Just do it.

- Make a list of treatment centers in your area.

- Order a copy of *Alcoholics Anonymous, Fourth Edition* (aka, the Big Book) online.

- Order a daily meditation book for people in recovery.

- Order *Twenty-Four Hours a Day* (the first meditation book for alcoholics).

- Read articles, pamphlets, or books on the subject of addiction and recovery.

- Read posts by drug abusers suffering health consequences.

- Read the Big Book.

- Say a prayer and meditate.

- Search online for an addiction medicine specialist.

- See if there is an addictions counselor in your neighborhood.

- Speak to your pastor, priest, or rabbi.

- Take an online assessment.

- Take advantage of your Employee Assistance Program (EAP).

- Talk to a trusted friend.

- Talk to your family doctor (many doctors hear these issues on a weekly basis).

- Talk to your spouse or closest loved one about your concern.

- Talk to a therapist.

- Visit the National Institute on Drug Abuse (NIDA) website (www.drugabuse.gov) and read the latest research about addiction.

- Write down a list of baby steps you can take to get help (pick some from this list).

- Write down in a journal or notepad why you think you might need help.

- Write down what you want your life to look like.

- Write down what your life looks like.

- Write down your alcohol/drug history.

The most important thing to do, now that you've read this book, is to put it down and get help. Procrastination is not an option. Right now, promise yourself. As you have this book in one hand, dial with the other hand. Let's make this first move together.

So whether you take that baby step in a doctor's office; with a counselor, a friend, or a stranger at an AA meeting; via an online test; or by having a clinical diagnostic evaluation, take the next baby step and act on the recommendations.

When you finally confront the facts about this disease in your life, take the first steps and keep walking in a positive direction. I wish you every bit of success. I'm including at the end of this book (see page 243) a few helpful websites and phone numbers for those of you who are brave enough, or concerned enough, or frightened enough, or blessed enough to take that first step. God bless you and good luck.

— TAKEAWAYS —

» Everyone's path into recovery is unique.

» Inpatient and outpatient treatment, AA or NA, and recovery literature are all common paths into recovery.

» We don't have to wait until we hit rock bottom to get help.

» Addiction provides us with an unlimited number of excuses for why we can't begin a recovery program.

» Taking even a small baby step can set a miraculous string of events into motion.

———

I WAITED UNTIL I was 54 years of age, forced by the consequences in my life to finally feel sick and tired of being sick and tired, to give up my fight and break through my procrastination. At that moment in time, the weight of the world fell off my shoulders. I felt an enormous sense of relief, like how it feels to clean out the mess in a closet or garage after looking at it for 2 or 3 years, only multiplied a millionfold.

I completed my treatment at the Betty Ford Center in 13 weeks (or 90 days) and returned home knowing something incredible had happened. I eagerly connected with friends who I knew had this disease, and many of the patients I had sent to treatment over the years welcomed me into the program without judgment.

And a different kind of magic began appearing in my life. In 2005, Mike Neatherton, president of the Betty Ford Center, told me of a new program being developed for health care professionals and offered me the opportunity to head it up as Physician Director. This was music to my ears. My mother was gone and my son, Aram, had married and moved south. My ties to Vermont were loosening, and I felt drawn to drink from the waters that I had found in treatment. Every cell in my body screamed for more, and I wanted to pay it forward by helping others still suffering. Without a moment's hesitation, I loaded up a moving van in Vermont and traveled cross-country to Palm Desert, California.

I still, however, had unfinished business in Vermont. I still had to provide urine samples at random intervals for the Vermont Practitioner Health Program, the monitoring program in which I had enrolled. I would trudge back on a monthly basis to be monitored—I had a 5-year contract to fulfill. I was also trying to operate my sports medicine and family practices, but my heart was truly in addiction medicine back in the desert.

There were many miracles around that time. When I traveled to the Betty Ford Center as a guest lecturer and alumnus, eager to share my story with others, I had the opportunity to meet and court my beloved Nicolette and to get to know her extraordinary family. Eventually, we married. I got my boards in addiction medicine and began my full-time job at the Betty Ford Center. And so began my new life. One day at a time.

I've not had a drink or drug since that time. Although I did require some medication during subsequent surgeries—a hip replacement and several abdominal procedures—my experiences confirmed that, with expert involvement, one can get through these medically necessary procedures without jeopardizing sobriety. And I have never had to white-knuckle it.

There, but for the Grace of God, go I.

CHAPTER 14

EMOTIONAL SOBRIETY AND ADVANCED RECOVERY TOPICS

"I tried to drown my sorrows, but the bastards learned how to swim, and now I am overwhelmed by this decent and good feeling."

—FRIDA KAHLO

WHEN I WORK with clients, I often use a piece of chalk and a black-board to explain how those of us with the disease of addiction usually approach our diagnosis. First, I put a tiny dot on the blackboard and then back up a few feet. I then act as if an oncologist is right next to me explaining that this dot is my chest X-ray. "Harry, that lesion you had on your arm should have been biopsied because now I see it on your chest: malignant melanoma."

After that whammy of a statement, I don't hear anything else. I illustrate this to my client by moving closer to the dot, my nose now up against the blackboard. At this point, my vision and hearing block out everything but the fact that I have cancer. My whole life is suddenly wrapped around this diagnosis—this white dot. I will do anything I need to do to get this out of my life. I quickly agree to get 6 months of therapy, radiation treatment, and to visit the oncologist office weekly, monthly, and then bimonthly.

After 5 years of treatment, I'm in a state of cure or remission. The dot has gotten smaller and is in my rearview mirror. I'm aware that the dot is ever present and that I need to follow my cancer recovery regimen daily or the disease could return, but my life encompasses more than my diagnosis now.

To show clients how differently most people respond when they learn they have the disease of addiction, I go in a back corner of the room, against the wall, as far away as I possibly can from the dot on the blackboard. I then exclaim, "That's not me!"

While the cancer patient builds their life around getting better, just the opposite happens when people get a diagnosis of addiction. Rather than embrace the solution, we deny the problem. But as we slowly start to do the program—go through the Steps, surrender, get some acceptance—we begin walking toward the dot.

As time goes by, say, after 10 years, our notion of sobriety should be bigger than it was when we were first diagnosed. We should, in other words, be closer to the dot. We have learned how deadly the disease is and how it affects everything in life. The hope is that the following year, we'll be even closer to the dot, and with 20 years of recovery under our belt, our face will be flat against the blackboard, where we keep it for good.

A high-quality recovery from addiction takes time and diligence. The more we grow in recovery, the more wrapped up we become in the diagnosis and in our efforts to get better. The dot is never in our rearview mirror but right under our nose.

In this chapter, I introduce you to emotional sobriety and advanced recovery topics. This is the maintenance stage of recovery we talked about in Chapter 4. In this phase of recovery, we are beyond learning "how to stop" and "how to cope." Here we learn "how to live." It's an exciting phase of recovery and something to which we can look forward. This final stage of recovery opens up great new horizons in our relationship with self and others. We become a better partner, parent, coworker, and citizen—a better person overall.

Continuing to work on recovery, even when we have no desire to drink or use, keeps our focus on the dot on the blackboard. And that's where we want to be. Being fully immersed in recovery puts us in a state of being "happy, joyous, and free" much of the time.

EMOTIONAL SOBRIETY

Being sober goes beyond abstinence or the physical act of not drinking or using. There's also a large emotional component to recovery. Without alcohol or drugs to "drown our sorrows," we start feeling the emotions we buried while actively using. Some of these feelings can be overwhelming. Any of these feelings can be excuses to return to our drug of choice.

Emotional sobriety is accepting how we feel at any given moment, whether we want to feel that way or not. Although this work begins the moment we first put down our drink or drug, it's a lifelong, day-by-day practice that we continue to refine for the rest of our lives.

Achieving emotional sobriety means being at peace with how we feel, no matter how we feel. It's understanding that it's okay not to be happy all the time. Taking it one step further, it means staying sober no matter how we feel. It's a commitment to using tried and true principles and practices on a daily basis to stay sober while also being fully alive—experiencing life's ups and downs without resorting to alcohol or other drugs to block or enhance our feelings.

Because feelings are always with us, our emotional sobriety work never ends. Being in touch with how we feel can help us to heal. And so emotional sobriety is something we must always work on. I would go so far as to say it is the goal of recovery.

The trick to achieving emotional sobriety is not to judge how we feel at any given moment but to accept it—and then express it maturely by taking responsibility for how we feel.

For instance, if we're frustrated with the slow driver we're stuck behind on the highway, we could express it the old way—by yelling expletives and slamming our hands against the steering wheel, increasing the anxiety of everyone in the car with us. Or, we can express our frustration maturely. Doing that is a process.

A mature expression of frustration might look something like this:

- Acknowledgment: We acknowledge, maybe even voice out loud, that we are frustrated with the slow driver.

- Curiosity: We become curious about why we are frustrated. Is it because we will be late for an appointment and really should have left the house sooner? Is it because we have no tolerance for drivers who can't at least go the speed limit and probably shouldn't have their license?

- Compassion: We bring compassion and kindness into the picture—first toward ourselves and then the driver.

The truth is we should have left the house earlier and given ourselves time to allow for heavy traffic (or slow drivers). We didn't leave earlier because we snoozed the alarm after having a restless night's sleep. But we did our best. If we are late, we can take responsibility for being late by apologizing. The slow driver may have reasons for not going the speed limit that we are unaware of. Maybe he is preoccupied with thoughts about a loved one in the hospital or a big presentation he's about to give to a new client. It's not our place to judge the driver and take our frustrations out on him by blaming him for our predicament. We take responsibility for the possibility that we'll be late. But we still have a good chance of making it to our appointment on time. After all, speeding only takes a few minutes off our commute.

Achieving a state of emotional sobriety leaves us feeling serene—calm, unruffled, grounded, and balanced. We accept life on life's terms. We are imperfect and unafraid to express that truth. We possess a strong faith in our recovery and can turn to the Twelve Steps to help us be mindful of any character defects that interfere with our emotional sobriety.

ADVANCED RECOVERY TOPICS

In the following paragraphs, I introduce 16 common issues that can stall recovery and make us feel as if we've hit a wall. I pose these topics as questions—as food for thought. Working on these issues can catapult our recovery progress.

Not everyone is ready to deal with these topics right off the bat. Some people require a good solid recovery foundation. Early on in our addiction, when we're focused on not drinking or using, it can be overwhelming to deal with these concerns. Some of them are complicated.

As we spend more time in recovery, the brain has a chance to heal. As cognition improves, our ability to deal with these topics improves. I will let you be the judge of whether you are ready to work on any one of them in early recovery or whether you want to wait until you've gone through all the Twelve Steps or have a solid foundation of recovery. Just know that it is perfectly fine to wait.

To fully enjoy the gifts of recovery, we must at least be mindful of these topics and, when ready, address them with the help of the Twelve Steps, a sponsor, or other support. Dr. James West, cofounder of the Betty Ford Center and its first medical director, said that the answer to any problem can be found in the Twelve Steps. While I encourage you to consider using the Steps to deal with any of the following advanced recovery topics, I acknowledge that some of you will prefer to seek alternative methods, either through talk therapy, religion, Buddhism, or other groups that promote abstinence-based recovery. I encourage you to find recovery in the way that works best for you.

Each of the questions below concerns an advanced recovery topic. When you feel ready, ask yourself the following questions:

Do I live one day at a time?

Character defects (Chapter 5) often emerge when we bite off more than we can chew and get overwhelmed. Remember the slogan One

Day at a Time (ODAAT). Living ODAAT helps us to savor recovery. We're able to realize the promises of recovery that are yet to unfold and see a glimmer of hope every day.

What is the quality of my surrender?

Recovery depends on our ability to surrender to the disease of addiction every day. Surrender means we cease fighting anything or anyone—even alcohol and other drugs. Surrendering puts us in a neutral position where we are safe and protected. We get a daily reprieve from the "dry drunk," or behaving as poorly as we did when we were using, even though we are no longer using. We get a daily reprieve from our defects of character, which can pop up like mushrooms on the lawn. The Twelve Steps, as we learned in Chapter 5, help us to confront character defects.

Do I try to be humble whenever possible?

In humility, we never miss the opportunity to get smaller. True recovery is the product of humility, which emerges from practicing a conscious and spiritual life. The Tenth Step helps us to maintain the attitude and actions that protect our gift of recovery—the gift we must share at every opportunity.

Have I accepted that addiction is a powerful, fatal brain disease?

Learning how to live requires accepting not only that we have a problem with addictive substances but that it is a potentially deadly problem. Addiction is a chronic brain disease with psychosocial consequences. Addiction is a fatal disease that requires that recovery be our first priority. There's an AA saying that the disease is doing push-ups in the parking lot waiting for us to have a relapse. Unless we have the notion that the disease can get more and more powerful, we'll never respect it enough. We let our guard down and it shows up unannounced.

We don't need to be paranoid, but a few simple practices each morning keep recovery front and center stage in our lives and the disease at bay. Every morning we can do the following:

1. Admit we're an alcoholic/addict and pray.

2. Embrace the notion that whatever we did yesterday got us to bed safe and sober. Be grateful we had a day without alcohol. Know that if we do what we did yesterday, there's a good chance we'll be safe.

3. Practice Step 3: Decide to turn our will and our lives over to the care of God as we understand Him.

Have I defined my addiction system and built a recovery system that includes those closest to me in my program?

An addiction system is how we defend (and others support) our drinking or drug use. It's the doctor who works in the ER for 12 to 15 hours. He gets through his shift by taking amphetamines. He works until midnight and has to go back again in 12 hours, so he takes Ambien and alcohol. After work he stops at the bar, where he's well known. He provides free health care for all his bartenders and never pays for a drink. Everybody says, "Doc, you deserve it. It's on the house." That's an addiction system.

A recovery system acknowledges that an addiction system exists and takes steps to mitigate its power. The doctor, for instance, might arrange to work shorter shifts or give his spouse instructions for what to do if he is not home at a certain hour.

Is my life driven by positive or negative spiritual principles?

In *Finding Your Moral Compass,* counselor and author Craig Nakken talks about how human beings are part animal and part spirit. The animal side of us is driven by instinct, while the spirit side is driven by spiritual principles, which can be positive (love, truth) or negative (hate, lies). When we embrace positive spiritual principles, we are enriched. Negative spiritual principles give us a false sense of control and go against our conscience. In this state we are lying to ourselves, which leaves us feeling anxious and prone to relapse. For more on how to identify when you are operating from negative spiritual principles and how to put positive spiritual principles first, I highly recommend reading *Finding Your Moral Compass.*

Is there room for other opinions in my life?

Being open-minded is a sign that we're willing to grow. Do we allow plenty of room for other people and their opinions in our life, with healthy, flexible, and adjustable boundaries? Everything is not about us, and we are not always right. Other people matter.

Do I actively choose faith or insanity every day?

A definition of insanity often attributed to Albert Einstein is: "Doing the same thing over and over again and expecting different results."

Doing the same thing over and over again expecting the same result is called faith. Actively choose faith over insanity every day.

Have I discovered other addictions in my quest to be sober from alcohol and other drugs?

Codependency (addiction to people), workaholism, overeating, and compulsive gambling and shopping are different expressions of addiction. If we've replaced one addiction for another, we haven't gotten to the spiritual root of the problem. We've just switched gears.

What are my strategies to ensure mental and physical health?

Good health requires that we maintain a mindful balance of relationships, emotions, and nonchemical methods to deal with stress and anxiety. What are my social connections all about, and do they promote recovery? What behavioral therapies do I use? Do I eat a nutritious diet? Do I stay active? As I get older, do I confront changes in cognitive abilities with evidence-based strategies to avoid problems with memory, speed of processing, cognition? Don't underestimate the importance of brain health. Many people relapse when they start to experience cognitive decline.

Do I make sure I'm held accountable for my behavior?

Pulse, respiration, blood pressure, and temperature are four essential vital signs we use in the medical field to assess a person's health. For addiction, I add a fifth vital sign: accountability. Accountability requires accepting responsibility for our actions. And it means we do what we say we will do. Without accountability, we tell ourselves we can do whatever we want whenever we want—even drink or use.

Am I prepared for the possibility that I might slip?

Being prepared for challenges to recovery is the best way to protect your recovery—your investment in you. Leave little to chance. Reveal your relapse prevention plan. Know that your family may contribute to your demise: "Do you really have to go to a meeting? You're doing so well!" Involve your therapist. The fear of losing family or a license does not keep you sober. The consequences of continuing to use must be greater than the fear of stopping.

Do I continue to embrace the four movements needed for a positive recovery?

The four movements required in recovery are: fear to trust, dishonesty to honesty, self-pity to gratitude, and resentment to acceptance.

Do I understand the four paradoxes of the program?

The four major paradoxes are: Surrender to win. Give it away to keep it. Suffer to get well. Die to live.

Do I have a 20-hour-a-day schedule?

Some fundamental recovery tools cannot be overlooked. We do best when, on most days, we devote 1 hour for a Twelve Step meeting,

1 hour for prayer and/or meditation, 1 hour for physical self-care, 1 hour for fun and time to journal and to talk to others. This leaves us 20 hours for sleep, work, and family.

TRAITS OF SUCCESS

Successful, long-term recovery looks something like this:

- We are connected spiritually to a recovery program and sponsorship and having friends in recovery.
- We live a balanced lifestyle 20 hours a day.
- We make recovery the most important focus in our life.
- We know and practice the antidote for relapse: gratitude, dignity, and self-respect.
- We comprehend that recovery is not for the lazy.

SIMPLE . . . BUT NOT EASY

Recovery is often described as "peeling an onion." It's a process with many layers. As we get deeper into recovery, we'll find new issues to address. It's important to understand what the most common threats to long-term recovery are so we are able to recognize them if and when they surface. Recognizing these new layers enhances not only our recovery but our entire life!

Recovery is simple, but it is not easy. Rather, it is hard work. But it is worth it. The rewards of working through some of these issues are many—including the "decent and good feeling" we find ourselves enjoying more and more often.

CHAPTER 15

THE PROMISES AND THE TWELVE TRADITIONS

"Courage is fear that has said its prayers."

—DOROTHY BERNARD

ALONG WITH THE Twelve Steps, the Big Book gives us 12 promises, commonly referred to as the Promises. The Promises tell us what we can expect if we follow the Twelve Step program. Those of us who have adhered to the Twelve Steps know that the Promises are real. They come true when we work the program.

There is no mention of alcohol or drugs in any of the Promises. Instead, they stress freedom from the bondage of addiction. The primary lesson here is that sobriety does make promises, and it keeps them.

THE PROMISES

PROMISE ONE: **"We are going to know a new freedom and a new happiness."** Through surrender and acceptance, we find a new freedom. We recognize the reality of our addiction, and our new freedom is from the burden of fighting a battle that we never seemed able to win. Happiness and peace of mind in sobriety replace the false joys of addiction. Joy and laughter replace despair, and our new choices lead to spiritual growth. This first promise brings freedom, honesty, gratitude, humility, faith, and trust.

PROMISE TWO: **"We will not regret the past nor wish to shut the door on it."** This second promise tells us that all of the difficulties we have had in the past—trouble with the law, trouble with relationships, trouble with finances—will serve a purpose for us and for others, lessons to be learned and taught. Regardless of the depths to which we've plummeted while in our disease, no experience can be too awful to help another alcoholic or addict.

With this promise, our regrets subside and our gratitude increases. Freedom from guilt over past deeds and learning from our old mistakes allow us to use our memories as tools for growth and relapse prevention. Protection from complacency and carelessness comes when we keep our experiences new and green, always remembering our last drunk rather than our last drink and avoiding the pitfalls of euphoric recall, a process where we tend to pretty up our past to make it more acceptable and palatable in the present.

PROMISE THREE: **"We will comprehend the word *serenity*, and we will know peace."** Here we get to define *serenity* for what it means to us: maturity, gratitude, acceptance, awareness, and brotherly love. Integrating the principles of the Steps into our lives brings us contentedness, knowing that all we need will be provided. We will know peace, no longer burdened by the struggles of our will against that of a Higher Power.

As we discard our character defects, our shame disappears. As we act with honesty and integrity, we become whole. We feel the difference on the inside. Regardless of what is going on around us, we carry a strong inner peace with us. We are no longer drinking or drugging to kill pain. Sobriety uses past pain for our emotional growth and healing. Indeed, the goal of recovery is attaining emotional sobriety and preventing relapse. Our disease is denial. Recovery is based on acceptance, surrender, courage, and wisdom. So we will comprehend the word *serenity* as gratitude for what we have. It is active and constructive, and it creates a climate for growth. It makes forgiveness possible.

PROMISE FOUR: **"No matter how far down the scale we have gone, we will see how our experience can benefit others."** Our experience has value, and when we share, we see similarities with others who suffer. And it is through our common welfare that recovery takes shape. This ability to share with one another allows high-bottom and low-bottom addicts and alcoholics to identify with each other. The person who experiences absolute incomprehensible demoralization can share his experience and prevent someone else from having to go that low himself. With true identification, that kind of crash is unnecessary. Honesty and sincerity are key elements to relating to the still-suffering alcoholic or addict.

PROMISE FIVE: **"That feeling of uselessness and self-pity will disappear."** Feelings of uselessness and self-pity are self-centered thinking. We no longer have to concentrate on being the worst of the worst or the best of the best. We can concentrate more on our brother and our sister in recovery, and we'll know quickly that all of our experiences can be of use to another who still struggles.

We become worthwhile. We are given our self-respect and rediscover our purpose. Gratitude and humility give us a second chance at life.

PROMISE SIX: **"We will lose interest in selfish things and gain interest in others."** As people-pleasers, our motives were selfish. We acted for material and emotional rewards. Drugs and alcohol drove our ego to a false sense of power and importance. In recovery, we naturally move from connecting with our chemicals to connecting with others. Generously sharing ourselves is the answer—random acts of kindness with no expectations of return. Remember, we can do together what we can't do alone. By sharing, we rid ourselves of pride, self-righteousness, envy, jealousy, and resentment.

PROMISE SEVEN: **"Self-seeking will slip away."** Our motives have changed. We do not need to be loved by others to feel validated. Our grandiosity and self-centeredness will no longer be needed to protect our right to drink and drug. Self-made successes worship their creators—their egos—rather than their Higher Power. Humility quietly enters where we become teachable in this promise. We truly begin to clean our own house. We do not need to invest ourselves in the outcome; we simply do the work for the betterment of the whole.

PROMISE EIGHT: **"Our whole attitude and outlook on life will change."** We begin to trust that our needs will be met. We honestly go about our day with boundaries and limitations that we've defined for ourselves, keeping our priorities (i.e., our recovery) front and center in all that we do. We begin to accept life on life's terms, and we stop blaming others. We no longer seek others to validate our worth. We know our limitations and our potential. Our approach changes from hostile and negative to positive and friendly. Self-loathing gives way to self-esteem. Our one-day-at-a-time approach—living in the now—prevents us from experiencing guilt from the past and fear of the future. We feel grateful at the end of the day, and we express it through love and service.

PROMISE NINE: **"Fear of people and economic insecurity will leave us."** We realize that fear comes from within and that we, not others, are our own worst enemy. Sobriety decreases fear, envy, low self-esteem, resentment, reactions, and frustration. In the Fellowship, we lose loneliness and begin experiencing feelings for others. Love and sobriety, true caring and sharing, and acting with and for others in recovery form the basis of our spiritual awakening. Simply having financial security and freedom from fear means that we will receive what we need, not always what we want.

PROMISE TEN: **"We will intuitively know how to handle situations that used to baffle us."** We will not let ourselves get involved in areas that are none of our business, and where it is our business, we bow to the will of our Higher Power, trusting and praying for a solution. We will suddenly realize that these promises will come true by simply living a right life and doing the next right thing. Coping becomes easier. "If it ain't broke, don't fix it." We learn that time is the great teacher—patience, "easy does it," "one day at a time." This promise guarantees spiritual growth through humility and acceptance.

PROMISE ELEVEN: **"We will suddenly realize that our Higher Power is doing for us what we could not do for ourselves."** When using, we could not accept God's time schedule for us. Grandiosity said, "I can do it alone. I don't need any help." Our ego fought to retain control. In this promise, we realize that once we know the will of our Higher Power, it becomes our responsibility to carry it out.

PROMISE TWELVE: **"The promise of sobriety will always materialize if we work for it."** Our recovery evolves through effort and action. How quickly or slowly we grow depends on the quality and quantity of work we do. Following instructions in each step of our spiritual growth and being patient enough to find true solutions and not just other problems in disguise are the keys. We must follow a well-worn path, one step at a time. If the definition of insanity is doing the same thing over and over and getting the same result, then faith can work the same way and provide a positive outcome. The Promises come true—sometimes quickly, sometimes slowly—but they do come true.

THE TWELVE TRADITIONS

I include the Twelve Traditions in this book because they are so important to understanding why the Twelve Step program has helped so many and can help you. The traditions are 12 practical principles, or guides, that serve to protect and preserve the Fellowship from corruption and other controversial behaviors that could affect or even destroy the organization as a whole.

History has recorded the rise and fall of many political, religious, and social programs. For instance, the Washingtonians, a 19th-century temperance society advocating total abstinence, outlived their usefulness and stopped growing as an institution when they invited controversy by involving themselves with self-promotion and arrogant exhibitionism. They competed with other organizations and were preyed upon by politicians. Although they grew massive in numbers in only a few short years, ultimately, they disappeared.

In 1948, Bill W. wrote, "The individual is subjected to glorification, consuming ambition, exhibitionism, intellectual shyness, money, and refusal to admit mistakes." The Twelve Traditions are really Twelve Steps for the group. So far, these basic principles have worked to keep Alcoholics Anonymous and its offshoots constructive, respectable, and transparent organizations.

TRADITION ONE: **"Our common welfare should come first; personal recovery depends upon AA unity."** The program's security is founded on the principles of humility. Compliance is a matter of individual conscience, not judgment. We set aside petty ambitions, and—as a group—concern ourselves with the welfare of the group as a whole. Of course, *drugs and alcohol will discipline us* if we backslide from this mission.

TRADITION TWO: **"There is but one ultimate authority—a loving God as He may express Himself in our group conscience."** Like the individual, the group—through its thoughts, experiences, conscience, and Twelve Step work—recognizes its own character defects. Each group is different. Experience leads to recognition of these problems. This leads the group to change appropriately in the sight of these misgivings. When experience and change proved to be for the betterment of the group as a whole, these experiences were written down as AA Traditions. Group conscience will always prove more favorable for the group's welfare than the will of any individual.

TRADITION THREE: **"The only requirement for AA membership is a desire to stop drinking."** No one is excluded; we cannot rule out any applicant. After 10 years of experience, the original groups of AA developed rules of membership. They were found to be so stringent that newcomers could barely qualify. This tradition is based on the knowledge that AA as a whole can hardly be harmed by any individual regardless of lifestyle or background. Each individual may be different, but no one is excluded. This also is a tradition that

allows for special interest groups—women, men, gay, straight, doctors, pilots, attorneys—to organize where specific life circumstances
are used to qualify. But these attendees are first and foremost AAs in
the general membership.

TRADITION FOUR: "**Each AA group should be autonomous
except in matters affecting other groups as a whole.**" Though autonomous, we are part of a bigger whole with a common welfare. Here,
each group is free to work out its own customs, formats, meeting
lengths, and so forth. Like the individual, the organization is a living
entity. Implicit in our singleness of purpose, we are constantly threatened as a society by our own set of character defects. One group
might have an inflated ego, which might cause adverse effects on the
larger Fellowship. A renegade group may appear to the public to be
representative of the Fellowship as a whole. It is dangerous when a
group strays from the path. Like Step Four, Tradition Four requires
an inventory of group action to avoid breaking any tradition.

TRADITION FIVE: "**Each group has but one primary purpose—
to carry its message to the alcoholic who is still suffering.**" Simply
put, we help others: "I am responsible when anyone, anywhere,
reaches out for help. I want the hand of AA to always be there, and
for that, I am responsible." *We learn to carry the message and not
the mess.* We may help others individually and judiciously with finding work, shelter, and finances, but not as a group or an agency. We
offer the hope that an alcoholic can recover in this organization.
Other agencies that are our friends take on the responsibility of public education about alcoholism. Boundaries need to be set for this
relationship.

TRADITION SIX: "**An AA group ought never endorse, finance,
or lend the AA name to any related facility or outside enterprise, lest
problems of money, property, and prestige divert us from our pri-**

mary purpose." We have no outside affiliations. Counselors may wear two hats but never at one time. In other words, they may be counselors and work with alcoholics or addicts, but in the rooms of AA they can be alcoholics themselves and do not ply their trade in the meetings. AAs who have formed outside enterprises must keep AA and Twelve Step out of their name. Our policy with these agencies is cooperation and not affiliation. We may welcome clinicians who refer to a group or take a meeting to an institution, so there is a relationship capability built into this tradition, guided by highly demarcated boundaries.

TRADITION SEVEN: "Every group ought to be fully self-supporting, declining outside contributions." Although we have expenses, our membership provides enough for our primary purpose, so we do not put our hands out, as Bill W. said, "like we did when we were drinking." There is a $1,000 limit on annual contributions and wills. No one person may carry more influence than another. We keep a prudent reserve for important expenses. Here we have equal access to AA services and activity.

TRADITION EIGHT: "AA should remain forever nonprofessional, but our service centers may employ special workers." This tradition tells us work is work. We pay for it honorably and with humility. Our Twelve Step work is free, and the grace of our Higher Power pays us for that. No member of AA can accept payment for carrying the message face-to-face. People in the AA Central Office are employees and work to maintain meeting schedules and memberships and to facilitate detoxification. They operate phone lines for Twelve Step calls; they help keep the message pure and in tune with the group conscience. Our General Service Office has become too big for volunteer labor. We pay them well to keep us humble. We do not expect free work for "the privilege of working in AA."

TRADITION NINE: "AA, as such, ought never be organized; but we may create service boards or committees directly responsible to those they serve." We have special opportunities to serve others face-to-face. We need to carry our message and keep our simplicity. We need organization, not chaos, to carry the message. The essence of this program is spiritual simplicity. We respond to the cry for help.

TRADITION TEN: "Alcoholics Anonymous has no opinion on outside issues; hence the AA name ought never be drawn into public controversy." Here we *keep it simple,* keep it pure, and avoid outside distraction. Simply put, we try to mind our own business; we do not proselytize.

TRADITION ELEVEN: "Our public relations policy is based on attraction rather than promotion; we need always maintain personal anonymity at the level of press, radio, and films." There is no individual glory. We are talking of personal anonymity here. AA as a whole needs to educate the public of its existence, but no one individual can represent the organization. There is too much danger that too many character defects in one individual could injure the organization as a whole.

TRADITION TWELVE: "Anonymity is the spiritual foundation of all our traditions, ever reminding us to place principles before personalities." Here we humbly acknowledge our dependence on a Higher Power. Anonymity and humility are intricately related. We are not taking credit for our own or another's sobriety. These are gifts. True humility puts our self-respect on a solid base of truth rather than false pride. This reminds us that we recover through the Fellowship, not on our own. There are no big shots.

Let's look at the Twelve Traditions summarized in the spirit of simplicity:

1. We are not alone; we are united as a Fellowship.

2. No big shots, no bosses, just God as we understand Him.

3. No one is excluded. We cannot rule out any applicants.

4. Each group is autonomous and part of a larger whole devoted to our common welfare.

5. Our primary purpose is to help others and carry the message.

6. We have no outside affiliations.

7. We support ourselves and do not ask for handouts.

8. Work is work; we pay for it honestly and with humility. Our Twelve Step work is free. For that, our Higher Power pays us.

9. We have special opportunities to serve others face-to-face; we need order to carry the message and keep our simplicity.

10. We keep it simple, keep it pure, and avoid outside distraction.

11. There is no individual glory.

12. We humbly acknowledge our dependence on a Higher Power.

EPILOGUE

"Forgiveness means giving up all hope for a better past."

—LILY TOMLIN

I'M DRIVING DOWN a one-way road in Wilmington, Vermont—the scene of the crime. I come to a little narrow bridge, one that only allows room for one car. Suddenly, I am there, nose to nose with a black, unmarked cruiser. Behind the wheel, now wearing his sergeant stripes, is the rookie cop. I know he recognizes me because when I get out of the car and walk over to him, he puts his hand on his gun and rolls down the window.

That's when I say, "Do you know who I am?"

He replies, "I remember you well."

"Well, I remember you well, too, and I have to tell you that you saved my life. I have to thank you for my arrest and to beg your forgiveness and make amends for all the things I thought I wanted to do to you. And I have to plead with you never to give up your convictions for an alcoholic like me. Do what you have to do. My family owes you, and I owe you. You have given me back some dignity and some integrity. I can walk with my head high today. It'll only last until tomorrow, and then I've got to pray it comes back into my life again. As for seeing you—I've been praying for that day and night."

It brought tears to both of us. I hear that story is told in the Vermont State Police Barracks during training for every new class that comes through. Or at least I hope it is.

HELPFUL RESOURCES

PHONE NUMBERS

Keep these numbers on hand throughout your recovery (or save them in speed dial) so help is always a quick call away.

Al-Anon: 888-4AL-ANON
Alcoholics Anonymous World Services: 212-870-3400
Families Anonymous: 800-736-9805
Narcotics Anonymous: 818-773-9999

ONLINE RESOURCES

The following websites contain useful information regarding alcohol and drug addiction and recovery. Alcoholics Anonymous (AA) and Narcotics Anonymous (NA) are Twelve Step groups for those suffering from addiction. Al-Anon, Alateen, Nar-Anon, and Families Anonymous are Twelve Step groups established for family members of those suffering from addiction. Visit any of these sites to locate meetings in your area.

al-anon.alateen.org
alcoholics-anonymous.org
drugabuse.gov
familiesanonymous.org
findtreatment.samhsa.gov

fourgenerations.org
na.org
nar-anon.org
recoverymonth.gov
samhsa.gov

INDEX

sponsors, 114, <u>115</u>, <u>116</u>, 174
Twelve Step Fellowship, 76, 117,
126–29, 163, 231, 236
Comparing to, vs. identifying with, 112,
122, 124
Consciousness. *See* Awareness
Consequences, in relapse prevention
plan, 164
Contacts. *See* Community of support
Contemplation stage, of change, 27
"Continental alcoholism," <u>29</u>
Control
vs. balance, 194–95
high-functioning addicts and, 39,
44, 49
relinquishing, 105, <u>205–6</u>
Coping, 66–67, 233
Cortisol, 7
Cough medications, 177
Courage, Twelve Step role, 80–82
Cover-up behavior, 39–41
Cravings
duration of, 65
neurology of, 8, 15, 154
planning for, 63–65
as spiritual quest, 173
Cross-addiction
awareness of, 50
defined, 167–69
excuses in, 170–71
factors in, 169–73
overview, 178–79
prevention of, <u>61</u>, 173–78
Culture
of recovery, 111–13, 128–29,
151–52
treatment and, 208
Cure, vs. treatment, 3–4, 59, 155,
233–34
Cycling, 60–62

D

Daily inventories, 90–91, 135, 138
Daily maintenance, 89–90
"Date rape" drugs, 188
Delirium tremens, 62
Denial
disclosure and, 48–50

in high-functioning addicts, 45, 53
precontemplation stage as, 27
regarding relapse, 148
stress and, 133
Twelve Step role, 77–78
Dental care, cross-addiction risks,
169–70, 175
Depressant medications, list of, 188
Despair, Twelve Step role, 78–79
Determination stage, of change, 27
Detoxification, supervision of, 47,
62–63, 186–87
Dextromethorphan (DMX), 178
Diabetes, 3
DiClemente, Carlo, 26
Digestive system, 9
Diphenhydramine, 172, 178
Disclosure, fear of, 48
Discussion meetings, 119
Disease
addiction as, xiii, 3, 15–16, 152,
206–7
choice lacking in, 15–16, 206–7
genetic factors, 6
shame and, <u>13</u>
treatment vs. cure of, 3–4, 59,
155, 233–34
Dishonesty, 85–86, 105
DMX, 178
Dr. Bob (AA founder), 85, <u>101</u>
Doctors. *See* Physicians
Dopamine
addiction role, 5–6, 8, 171
progressive cycle effects, 8
Drug use/addiction. *See also* Prescription
drugs; Street drugs
friends, perception of drugs as, 28–29
need satisfaction and, 102
statistics regarding, 30
D.T.'s, 62

E

Early recovery, 16, 64–65, 72–73,
94, <u>124</u>
Ecstasy, 188
Ego. *See* Self-interest
Eighth Step, 88–89
Eleventh Step, 91–92, <u>143</u>